Immune-System Activation

OTHER BOOKS BY JOHN SELBY

Therapeutic Massage
Visionetics
Powerpoint
Responsive Breathing
The See Clearly Book
The Visual Handbook
Finding Each Other

JOHN SELBY WITH
MANFRED von LÜHMANN, M.D.

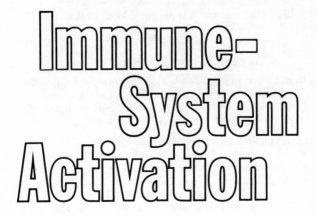

Immune-System Activation

PRACTICAL PROGRAMS
FOR MAXIMIZING YOUR
RECOVERY POTENTIAL

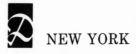

E. P. DUTTON　　NEW YORK

This book was first published in German in a slightly different version
by Droemer Knaur, copyright © 1987 by Droemersche
Verlagsanstalt Th. Knaur Nachf., München.
This English edition was first published by E. P. Dutton in 1989.

A NOTE TO THE READER: The ideas, procedures, and suggestions
contained in this book are not intended as a substitute
for consulting with your physician. All matters regarding
your health require medical supervision.

Published in the United States by E. P. Dutton,
a division of NAL Penguin Inc.,
2 Park Avenue, New York, N.Y. 10016.

Published simultaneously in Canada by
Fitzhenry and Whiteside, Limited, Toronto.

Originally published in West Germany in a German
translation as *Das Immunsystem aktivieren.*

Library of Congress Cataloging-in-Publication Data

Selby, John.
[Immunsystem aktivieren. English]
Immune-system activation : practical inner programs for maximizing
your recovery potential / John Selby with Manfred von Lühmann.
p. cm.
Translation of: Das Immunsystem aktivieren.
Bibliography: p.
Includes index.
ISBN 0-525-24693-2
1. Self-care, Health.   2. Immune system.   3. Mind and body.
I. Lühmann, Manfred von.   II. Title.
RA776.95.S44713 1989   88-18874
615.8′5—dc19   CIP

DESIGNED BY EARL TIDWELL

1 3 5 7 9 10 8 6 4 2

First American Edition

CONTENTS

Contents

Contents

FOREWORD

by Manfred von Lühmann, M.D.,
Director, Habichtswald Klinik für Ganzheitsmedizin

The primary question we have explored in this book is this: Can human beings actually help heal themselves when they fall ill or are injured? And if so, what practical guidance can help a person to optimize this inner-healing process?

It is well known by now, through the new science of psychoneuroimmunology, that the immune system is affected by various attutudes and emotional reactions in the human body. The hypothalamus does alter its functioning negatively based on the dominance of such emotions as grief, depression, chronic anxiety, and resentment, and positively through the increase of such emotions as joy, laughter, hope, and relaxed contentment.

The immune system itself is a vast network of interrelated organs and chemical messenger substances, along with nerve fibers in the bone marrow, the thymus gland, the spleen, and the lymph nodes. Each time we achieve a new breakthrough in our understanding of the immune system, we discover additional, unexpected dimensions to its influence throughout the body.

What John and I have been working on for a number of years now to determine is how a motivated person can consciously influence the functioning of this vast self-regulatory and healing system of the body when sickness does develop. We have observed that an important enhancement in self-healing seems to occur right when the patient realizes he or she has suffered enough, and is ready to reverse the condition. A certain learning has come about at deep levels of the personality, a turning point has been reached.

It is at this point that the programs outlined in this book can be of direct and impressive help in the healing process. When you can say, Yes, I want to heal myself; when you can say, Yes, I am ready to put my conscious energy into action to recover my vitality—at this point you can open this book and gain the professional guidance you may need to focus your mental and emotional energies properly, so as to help, rather than hinder, your recovery.

As a doctor, I want to point out that you will also want to benefit from medical treatment for your condition, while you work with the programs John will be teaching you. It is this combination of you and your medical support team that will make the difference in your recovery rate.

We do see definite evidence that your feelings and thoughts "talk" with the billions of defense cells in your immune system. Scientific understanding of how this communication between mind and body takes place is just beginning. But we can give a solid yes to such programs as John has developed with his wide range of medical and psychological colleagues.

Our purpose with these programs is not to offer false hope, but we do want to offer realistic hope where possible. It would not be fair to push all patients with terminal cancer or AIDS into a state of hoping for miraculous recovery, but there are always a few who, given the proper guidance for inner action, may be capable of such a reversal. And of course, the milder your condition, the better chance you stand of putting these inner-recovery techniques to successful application.

I have felt quite privileged that John turned to me so often during the last five years when he was seeking medical understanding of aspects of his immune-system activation programs. We have struggled long into many a night in our search for the correlation between what he understands as a therapist and I understand as a medical doctor. And I am very pleased that his book is now completed and available to the average person.

At my cancer clinic in Kassel we are using the same self-healing techniques that John teaches you in this book as an important tool in our overall recovery program. Every patient at the clinic has a copy of the book to work with, and every bed includes stereo equipment so that the patients can use John's cassettes (see Supporting Programs, pp. 178–81) whenever desired.

Together with their doctors, the patients choose particular techniques from the book to work with, and are given additional help in terms of personal counseling. After treatment the patients take their books and cassettes home with them to continue their self-healing meditations on their own. Preliminary reports have been very positive, and we feel it is a major step forward to have this book now available. I warmly recommend the entire immune-activation program you are about to delve into.

PREFACE

by John Selby

Looking back over history, we find that ever since the advent of modern medicine, doctors have been mystified by the wide variation in their patients' rates of recovery from illness. Two people of similar age and background may fall ill with the same disease, receive the same medical treatment, and yet have extremely different recovery rates.

Even more mystifying have been the recurring examples of people suffering from supposedly incurable diseases such as terminal cancer who have somehow managed to reverse their health condition and recover from the disease through their own internal power.

On a more common level, some of us may fall ill with the common cold or flu and recover quite quickly, while others continue to suffer for weeks or even months, remaining "under the weather" for long periods of time for no medically apparent reason.

Even when it comes to the healing of a broken leg or arm, two people of similar age and with similar treatment may demonstrate a very different rate of recovery. And in each person's lifetime, there are periods when we fall ill and can recover rapidly, whereas at other times we have great difficulty in throwing off the very illness that was easy to recover from earlier.

Recent medical research has finally documented scientifically what wise health observers have noted for centuries—namely, that a person's dominant emotional states, prevailing thought patterns and attitudes, diet and movement habits, and underlying spiritual atmosphere play vital roles in influencing one's rate of recovery.

What this means is that if your mental and emotional condition influences your healing potential, then, through consciously altering these internal variables, you can positively stimulate your immune system into more successful healing action.

The purpose of this book is to provide you with the practical techniques for accomplishing this inner triumph over whatever health problems might be plaguing you in the present moment, and to offer you a long-term program for maintaining good health in the future.

When our bodies are functioning in a healthy state, when we feel no physical symptoms of illness or injury, we tend to run through our days oblivious to the question of how human beings heal themselves.

But as soon as we find ourselves knocked down with one health affliction or another, then our entire perspective on the question becomes radically shifted, and we focus our attention seriously to the challenge of understanding the healing process, and of activating it within our own bodies.

My assumption as I am writing this book is that you are currently suffering from a particular illness or injury, and are seeking the most effective techniques for stimulating the recovery process that will bring you to good health again. Either that or you know someone who is sick and needing some extra encouragement and guidance in this positive direction.

The programs you will find in this book are the twelve most effective and practical techniques my colleagues and I have developed during the last two decades; these can be learned readily on your own and applied immediately to stimulate the functioning of your immune system. It is, after all, the relative performance of your immune system that determines your recovery rate, regardless of whether you are suffering from cancer or the common cold, from a broken arm or even the physiological and emotional traumas of a broken heart.

Whatever your personal health condition, medical evidence from many different sources has now made clear that a person's emotional condition, habitual thought patterns, attitudes, everyday routines, and spiritual balance as well, all play a vital role in determining the performance of the body's immune system. Even if your doctor is providing you with excellent medical help, your recovery rate can be seriously undermined if one of the above variables is interfering with your healing process.

As a therapist specializing in the relationship among physiological, mental, and emotional dynamics, I have struggled for quite a number of years to determine what practical techniques best facilitate the coordinated efforts of a person's healing mechanism. I have been lucky enough to do research work with a number of doctors and scientists, as well as exploring the more subtle dimensions of the psychological and spiritual factors in the healing process.

And what I want to do in this book is to present in a written format, which you can easily put to use without professional guidance, the most powerful techniques we have developed to date, for optimizing your recovery rate.

Such programs do not suddenly appear on the scene with no previous development. In fact, since time immemorial, human beings have been seriously studying the mysteries of the healing process, and observing certain definite factors that do influence a person's ability to throw off a sickness or injury and return to good health.

On one point there is almost universal agreement: the best path to optimum healing is a team effort, in which you receive the best support possible from medical and spiritual helpers, and at the same time take responsibility for doing everything possible to help yourself heal from the inside out—to resolve old emotional conflicts, expand constrictive attitudes, relax tense muscles, and create a more healthy inner spiritual atmosphere to encourage the biochemical healing processes that your immune system orchestrates.

I assume that you are already receiving adequate medical support for your health problem. What I want to offer is the guidance needed to bring about positive change at the levels of emotional, cognitive, intuitive, and spiritual health, so that these dimensions of your personality can augment, rather than thwart, your physiological healing process.

With each chapter, I am going to offer you a new inner technique for stimulating the recovery rate of your body. Some chapters will appear quite simple, teaching basic breathing and relaxation methods for tuning into your body at a deeper level. Other chapters will take you into more complex experiences such as balancing your emotional energies, gaining a new perspective on your personal past, and learning how to direct your mind's attention to stimulate the healing process in particular regions of your body. Still other chapters will offer suggestions on what foods to eat to optimize the healing process, what movements have proved most effective for stimulating immune functioning, and also what traditional spiritual exercises have demonstrated potent results in therapy applications.

Once you have explored all twelve of the techniques and felt their power in your own situation, you will have a full set of practical tools for helping yourself recover from your health condition, and also staying free of any health complications in the future.

You will notice that I have not presented a religious bias in this book. My aim has been to give each of you freedom to apply your particular religious beliefs to the techniques you learn, so that regardless of your religious preference, you can adapt these programs to your own personal belief system, and also work with your minister or spiritual guide, if you have one, to integrate these programs into your personal faith.

I do, however, very definitely see an underlying spiritual dimension to the healing process, no matter what theological interpretations you want to give this dimension. Ultimately there exists no separation among medical, psychological, and spiritual, when it comes to the functioning of the human organism. We are mysterious beings; no one fully comprehends how the healing process works; and I find it important to approach the healing experience with a sense of reverence and awe, even while we are putting to use very practical programs.

So with each new chapter, I hope you find opportunity through the techniques and meditations to grow on all four basic fronts of human experience: to expand your spiritual, emotional, and mental frontiers while also learning how to encourage the healing process at physiological levels in your body.

My hope is that doctors and nurses will find this book helpful in communicating to patients practical ways for working as a team in the recovery process. But I also hope that ministers and spiritual counselors can use this book with their clients as an essential link with the practical emotional and cognitive techniques that complement spiritual approaches to healing. In a word, I hope this book can become part of the teamwork needed to put together a well-rounded and successful recovery program.

There are a number of specific people who have directly contributed to the development of these twelve techniques I will be teaching you in this book, and I very much want to mention their names before we jump into the coming chapters. Dr. Williard Dalrymple and Professor Ralph Abraham of Princeton University, Dr. Humphrey Osmond of the New Jersey Bureau of Research in Neurology and Psychiatry, and the entire teaching staff at the San Francisco Theological Seminary, all were influential in guiding my studies and research into the relationship among the emotional, spiritual, and biochemical dimensions of the healing process.

In three quite different theological directions, Reverend William Gearhardt, Alan Watts, and Krishnamurti offered essential personal guidance into the more subtle aspects of the integration of mind, body, and spirit. And during my early years as a therapist, Charles Kelley, Dr. Alexander Lowen, and Dr. Francis Cheek showed me the psychological foundations on which many of the present healing programs are based.

More recently, during the five years I spent in Europe doing research work specifically related to the development of the programs in this book, I am deeply indebted to Professor Eduard Cartier of Zürich University, Dr. Hans Zimprick at the School of Medicine in Vienna, and Professor Manfred Henschel of the Free University in Berlin.

But I am especially thankful to my medical partner and mentor Manfred von Lühmann for his constant support and deep insights into the nature of realistic healing techniques. I initially met Manfred when he attended one of the seminars I was giving on my first lecture tour in Europe some six years ago, and I was immediately impressed both by his medical understanding of the functioning of the immune system, and by his ability to move beyond the limits of traditional medicine, to consider new approaches to enhancing the healing process.

To make a long story short, six months after beginning discussions with Manfred, I decided to move my practice from California to West Berlin, so that I could team up with Manfred and several other medical researchers in a shared practice. For the following four years, we were able to make great strides in determining which particular inner-healing techniques were most effective in helping clients recover quickly from a wide variety of medical problems.

We were also blessed with ample time to travel and meet with various experts in medicine and therapy; and it was from the combination of our practical work with clients and our participation in research programs being conducted in a number of countries that this present discussion has evolved.

At the same time that I am thankful to Manfred and the other advisers on this book, I do want to assume final responsibility for my success or shortcomings in communicating the programs and principles of healing included herein. Most of the techniques I will be teaching you have been developing in my work as a therapist for at least twelve or fifteen years, and although they are now ready to be offered to you for your personal use in helping yourself recover from your present malady, I do want to say that such techniques are in a constant state of development and evolution, and this book should by no means be seen as a final word on the subject.

As your doctor will certainly tell you, the question of immune-system activation, and of healing in general, remains a controversial and poorly comprehended phenomenon in medical science. But at the same time it should be remembered that human beings have been healing themselves since time immemorial, and it is no secret that some people are more successful with their recovery than others.

To end this Preface I want to say a beginning word about AIDS, to place this terrible immune-system disease in the broader context of the myriad health problems that are also immune-system related. Certainly the programs in this book should offer a powerful series of practical tools for AIDS-positive patients seeking realistic techniques for remaining free of AIDS-related health problems, and it is also hoped that these programs can help ease the symptoms if they have already developed.

However, in order to keep the focus of this book on the broader application of these recovery programs, I am going to reserve specific comment about AIDS applications until a later chapter in the discussion. It seems vital to place the AIDS problem in this wider context, so that all of us can gain a more universal understanding of the immune system's role in regaining and maintaining a positive health profile.

I hope that the programs presented here will serve all of you well, both in accelerating your present recovery rate and in helping you to remain free of health problems in the future. Best of luck, and God bless!

Immune-
System
Activation

1

THE BALANCE OF HEALTH

For almost all of us, our progression through life involves occasional bouts with illness and injury. And when we find ourselves caught in the grip of a sickness, be it a simple cold or a complex disease, we naturally ask ourselves why this has happened to us. We may know the general medical explanation for our condition, but we suspect that there are deeper dimensions to the deterioration of our health.

When I think back to the clients whom I have seen go through the process of recovering from an illness, what strikes me is that for most of them their illness was in many ways a blessing in their lives. Before the illness, there existed an imbalance somewhere inside them, and through the experience of the illness, this imbalance was detected, worked through, and transcended.

Both in ancient times and in the contemporary scientific era, illness has been seen as a basic imbalance in the system of the sick person. In ancient Greece, where modern medicine actually had its birth, the concept of *homeostasis* originated. It denotes the body's natural tendency to maintain an internal equilibrium, which enables all biological systems to function at an optimum level of health. The early Greeks noted that when the inner balance is lost, a mechanism within the body automatically goes to work to regain this equilibrium.

This same tendency of the body to maintain homeostasis is reflected in the functioning of the immune system. When a danger to the balanced functioning of the body is detected, an allout effort is launched to eliminate the threat to the healthy state of homeostasis.

The important addition to this picture that has developed in the last couple of decades, as I mentioned in the Preface, has been the inclusion of emotional and mental states of equilibrium as a determining factor in one's state of health. Of course, modern psychologists are not the inventors of this basic notion of balance and inner equilibrium. The great wisdom of ancient China, for instance, held the attainment of inner balance as key to all success in life. The American Indian tradition was also centered on the understanding of the necessity of balance in one's relationships both with nature, with other people, and one's inner self.

When caught in the throes of sickness or injury, we are wise to reflect on this question of balance and to be open to the possibility that we may need to go through some deeper transformation if we are to bring ourselves into a new state of inner balance. Illness, properly utilized, can be a passageway from one period of our life to a new period of better balance. Our basic attitude toward our present condition may determine much of the course of our illness.

If we contract against the sickness, judge it as purely negative, and refuse to learn from the experience and to grow, we tend to undermine our recovery potential. Even if we recover from the particular illness, our negative attitude toward the experience will predispose us to future health problems.

This does not mean we are at fault for creating our present health problem. Guilt is the last thing we need in our lives when we are ill, because it is almost always a negative emotion that pulls us even further off balance.

It is quite possible to assume responsibility for our next steps in life without taking on a burden of guilt for earlier steps. We all do our best at each point in life. If we have been unaware of certain aspects of life in the past, and created imbalances as a result, there is no cause for blame or guilt. Instead, we need to know that growth is possible, that old habits can be relinquished, that a more balanced state of mind and body can be attained.

Even if illness proves to be the doorway into that ultimate adventure of death itself, the attitude with which we approach the experience will determine the experience that comes to us.

Naturally, however, we fight against disease. We have a powerful life-force within that sustains us through our entire lifetime. The immune system will do all it can to orchestrate a recovery from illness. Unless our emotions, thought patterns, and old habits hold us in a constricted state that interferes with the functioning of the immune system, we have an excellent chance of regaining health and vitality.

A basic problem when we fall ill is our own anxious struggling against the disease itself. We generate stress through cognitive and emotional worrying, and this stress disrupts the biochemical processes that lead to recovery. In our very struggle to make ourselves healthy again, we may disturb the natural functioning of our bodies to generate renewed health.

Healing, as any doctor or nurse will testify, is something that cannot be forced. Healing seems to come quickest and easiest to those patients who finally accept their condition, surrender to the present moment, and relax into the healing process. With this surrender and acceptance, the body is free to fight the good fight, unhindered by the tensions and biochemical disturbances created by worrying, denial, muscular and glandular constrictions, and so forth.

I should perhaps mention at this point, in case you haven't heard the scientific news, that there have been great breakthroughs in artificially boosting the temporary functioning of the immune system. The pioneering research of Nobel Prize–winner Rita Levi-Montalcini of Italy and others have shown scientists how to manufacture a special group of growth-stimulating hormones that can boost the white-blood cell count in AIDS victims, for instance, and also cause enhanced growth of almost any other cells in the body.

The medical community is naturally very eager to have at its disposal such seemingly miraculous drugs for treating illness and injury. Certainly I am all in favor of the remarkable new era that is opening up with the artificial manufacturing of these "growth factors." In years to come, doctors will have available very powerful drugs for stimulating the immune system. But we must be very careful that we don't place all our hopes of healing on these chemical treatments to heal our superficial health problems quickly. These growth-factor drugs are in fact treating only the symptoms of a basic health imbalance. Such treatment will not cure the underlying causes of chronic illness.

My hope is that we can expand our medical success in treating symptoms of disease, and at the same time increase our sense of personal responsibility for regaining the basic homeostasis of our system, which is needed for lasting health. If we are seduced into placing all our trust in external treatments, we will ultimately be no better off with all the new immune-system-stimulation drugs than we were before them.

So without further hesitation, we should now begin to explore your own inner-healing potential. To begin this adventure, you might want to pause for a few moments right now before reading further. Put aside the book, close your eyes if you want to, and take a look at your present attitude about your ability to heal yourself from the inside out, with or without medical intervention. Take a look at your attitudes toward your present health condition, for instance, and see if you are ready to take the beginning steps toward regaining your optimum state of homeostasis. Take a few deep breaths, relax, and open yourself to whatever insights may come.

2

MIND-BODY INTEGRATION

When Manfred von Lühmann and I first started sharing our perspectives on the healing process, we found almost immediately a common observation about the state of mind of people who are ill or injured. This observation has become a foundation of the programs included in this book.

We had both noticed, among innumerable clients and patients who were ill, a strong tendency to spend most of the time either thinking about the future or lost in past reflections. Very little actual time was spent focused on the present moment. Thus very little conscious attention was being focused on the person's body right here, right now.

But in basic biological time, it is only right here, right now, within every ongoing moment, that the body actually heals itself. So a basic rule for encouraging immune-system activation is this: Hold your attention focused here in the present moment. Otherwise, with your conscious attention lost in the past or the future, you are doing yourself little good at all.

What is really meant by the present moment? Let's be very clear and straightforward about this, and not get lost in philosophical mind games. The present moment is, first and foremost, the perceptual reality within which your body lives. Your breathing, for instance, is totally in the present moment; by focusing on the actual movements you experience as you breathe, you can instantly tune into the here-and-now where healing takes place.

You can also tune into the beating of your heart as another primal way of coming fully into the present moment, because your heartbeat is located in the very center of the here-and-now.

A third reality orientation that defines the present moment is your body's constant interaction with the force of gravity. As you use your muscles to maintain your balance, you are bringing yourself into intimate contact with the present moment.

Beyond these three primary contacts, your senses are receiving information in the present moment and sending it to your brain in a continuous flow of the here-and-now around you and within you. Seeing, tasting, touching, hearing, smelling—these are your experiential anchors in the infinite sea of the present moment.

If, in fact, we have such strong natural inputs that help us to stay centered in the present moment, how is it that we lose ourselves so often in the past and the future?

Of course, it is the unique functioning of the human brain that makes habitual journeys into the past and future possible. Most animals lack this ability to reflect on their past and to project their consciousness into fantasies about what might come in the future. Likewise, most animals lack the cognitive ability to think in symbolic terms, to shift from perceptual reality to symbolic flights of mind.

Our remarkable ability to slip from the present into the past or future is neither positive nor negative. What is needed is a healthy interaction of all three dimensions of consciousness. When an imbalance exists, in this case inadequate time spent in the present moment, symptoms of the imbalance begin to manifest themselves in such things as health problems and accidents.

Until the age of four or five, all of us lived predominantly in the present moment, because we had not developed the mental capacity for past and future projecting. But at a certain point in our childhood, we made the remarkable discovery that we could escape the present moment through thought.

And it is at this point in our development, according to a growing number of professionals exploring cognitive links with chronic disease, that many of us established basic habits that, step by step, led to a personality structure that encourages disease in the body.

For many children, the present moment is a wonderful place to be. Life is full of adventure, love, sensory pleasures, and interpersonal rewards. But for other children, the present moment is often full of negative experiences, such as punishment, rejection by those close to them, and a wide assortment of fears and ugly situations. When they learn that they can escape the present moment by going back to remember a good experience, or through looking ahead to better times, or through fantasy flights where they create their own realities; when they discover the escape route of thought and fantasy, of memory and anticipation, then they regularly avoid the present moment.

After a time, a habit develops, a very powerful habit that can continue throughout life, even when times become better and there is no longer a need to escape the present moment. The mind unconsciously avoids the present moment, avoids direct experience of bodily functions, and, finally, avoids the mental focusing that helps activate the immune system during sickness.

And, of course, people who have little contact with

the moment-to-moment functioning of their own bodies are the very ones who fail to heed the warning signs of stress and imbalance in the body, and who tend to fall ill most often.

So we need to take an honest look at your own relationship with the ongoing present moment. Please don't think I am suggesting you start judging yourself; that would only be another mental process separating you from your body and the present moment. Instead, I am going to introduce you to the first step of the immune-system-activation program.

RECOVERY SESSION ONE

Regaining the Present Moment

This recovery session actually takes only a minute to do, so you will be able to do it quite often. And you can do it anywhere, anytime, without anyone's knowing you are doing a healing session at all. Like most extremely simple processes, it is also extremely powerful once you succeed in tapping its underlying potential. In fact, every recovery session that follows is built on the foundation of this first recovery session, so I hope you will open yourself to exploring it, step by step, during the next few days and perhaps weeks, and also make it a foundation of your living habits when you regain your health.

To regain the present moment, to hold your concentration to the here-and-now for a period of time, we need only follow the natural logic of the body itself.

1. First, turn your attention to your *breathing*. From your first moment after birth until your final moment before death, your breathing continues as the most powerful reminder of present-moment reality. And to the extent that you are aware of your breathing, you are aware of your whole body.

Although the idea of being aware of your breathing might seem simple, for most people the actual practice of watching the breathing can be very difficult to rediscover at first. So let me give you some ways to aid in this awareness process.

Rather than dealing with breathing as an abstract notion, notice that there are specific sensory experiences that come to you with every breath. *First, there is the sensation you can feel constantly of air flowing in and out your nose. Can you feel this right now?* Learning how to tune into this sensation regularly can be your primary beginning point for regaining the present moment. See if you can, over the next few days, gently develop and expand this awareness of airflow during inhales and exhales, and see where this awareness leads you.

Also, notice that you can feel the movements in your chest and abdomen as you breathe. This is another primal sensory input that expands your awareness of the present moment. To be aware of this feeling in your body, and the sensation of the air rushing in and out of your nose, both at the same time—is a great step into an encounter with your healing potential in itself.

To further aid in your breath-watching, you can say the word breathing *to yourself on every new exhale, to bring your cognitive mind into play in a way that directly helps integrate thinking and sensation—another great step forward. Try it:*

a. *feel the sensation of airflow in nose*
b. *feel the muscular movements while breathing*
c. *say "breathing"*

Once you have said *breathing* to yourself a few times, and experienced what you find when you turn your mind's attention in this direction, you can move directly on to the next step in this recovery session.

2. *With your next exhale, say the word* heartbeat *to yourself. Feel your heart's pulse somewhere in your body, at the same time that you remain aware of your breathing.*

Quite often, people have a block against feeling their heartbeat at all. Many anxieties can explain such a block. But you can move through this block by turning your awareness not just to the heart region, but anywhere in the body, because the pulse is actually felt throughout the body.

At some point, as you turn your attention to your pulse, you will suddenly feel an expanded awareness of your whole body, because your pulse is actually a whole-body phenomenon. Pause a moment to see if you experience this now:

○

3. *After saying the word* heartbeat *to yourself, you quietly inhale, and then on the next exhale, you say a third word,* balance. *By turning your attention, or rather by expanding it one step further, to your body's relationship with gravity, you come instantly into*

11

touch with both your muscles and your bones, which are constantly dealing with the challenge of balancing atop this spinning planet of ours.

Even if you are in bed on your back, you can move your body slightly and feel the effect of gravity on your muscles and bones. This direct sensation will lead you deeper into your awareness of your body as a whole.

4. You can now go a final step with body awareness, by saying whole body *on your next exhale. As you say this word to yourself, you should feel quite an unusual sensation. Normally, we tend to focus our attention to some point in our body, to a hand, or a foot, or a point of stimulation on the skin somewhere. But with this recovery session, we are doing something quite different with the mind's awareness of the body. We are striving toward a total awareness of the whole body at once.*

○

With these four basic words—*breathing, heartbeat, balance, whole body*—you have the beginning tools for reestablishing a deep relationship with your body. You also have a beginning way to bring yourself out of thought, out of chronic worrying about the future or mulling over the past, or drifting into fantasy. You have the technique for directing your attention where it is needed and freeing yourself from mental habits that get in the way of healing.

The question, of course, is whether or not you want to use this recovery session, this Present Moment meditation. My advice is this: If you enjoy doing the recovery session, wonderful, do it as often as you want to, many times a day. But if you don't want to, if something inside you resists this movement into the present moment, into awareness of the body, this too is fine. What you want to do instead is this: set aside four breaths, once an hour. And if you don't want to say the words to yourself with each breath, then just watch yourself *not* wanting to be aware of your body.

I know that many of you are going to be resistant to the very idea of turning your conscious attention to your body. After all, your body is your source of pain, of suffering, of inconvenience—of disease and injury. Why should you want to focus on this negative situation?

This is precisely the point of our present discussion: when we become ill, we tend to avoid the negative experience found in the present moment in our bodies. And through this avoidance, we take our potentially valuable conscious attention away from where it is needed.

If you find that you personally are doing this, as an unconscious habit, be gentle with yourself. A basic rule about consciousness is that you cannot force it to do anything. You need to work patiently with old habits of rejection and denial. My recommendation to return to your breathing once an hour, but not force yourself to do the recovery session, is the best beginning place for most people.

At the start of this section, I mentioned that many children avoid the present moment because it is associated with negative experiences in the past. Now, as you begin gently to turn your attention to the present moment consciously, you are likely to find once again (because you find yourself sick), that the present moment is not at all a nice place to be.

But look at what you do find with this Present Moment meditation: you find that you are still alive, which is after all something quite positive. Even when you relax and make no effort at all to breathe, you continue breathing, your life-force continues to encourage a positive attitude toward your condition. And even if you find your breathing and your heartbeat tense and constricted because of anxiety over your condition, or because of the pain you might feel, at least your heart is pounding regularly, sustaining your life moment to moment.

This doesn't mean I am a great believer in the power of positive thinking; I am not suggesting that you try to convince yourself how wonderful it is to be alive right now. I have been sick and I know how terrible it can feel at times to be conscious of the present moment.

But I also know that only through turning my attention to my breathing and heartbeat in the present moment have I managed at times of crisis to break free of the chronic tensions and apprehensions that were constricting my very life-force. And only when I focused on my breathing did it have a chance to alter its tense pattern.

In fact, with this first recovery session, you are gaining one of the most direct routes to accelerated recovery, because you are tapping one of the vital self-regulatory systems of the body. As long as you are unconscious of your breathing, it is a victim to old programming, and to the anxiety states generated by worry, and the like. But a seeming miracle happens when you turn your attention to your breathing. As you have perhaps already noticed, if you paused to try the Present Moment meditation just now, your breathing almost always changes when you turn your attention to it—and almost always in positive directions. When we turn to our breathing and find it constricted, we tend, in fact, to take a deep breath.

This is why, when a patient learns to do this Present Moment meditation successfully, a general relaxation happens throughout his or her system. And this movement into a more relaxed mental and bodily condition is usually the first step toward an enhanced recovery rate.

I have been doing this Present Moment meditation for quite a number of years now, and every time I do it, a new experience comes to me. The reason that one never tires of this meditation is that it always brings you into the present moment, and the present moment is always new, unique, surprising. Because the present moment has never happened before, it is an exciting time to live in—anything, including unexpected healing, can happen in the present moment, and nowhere else!

Without further words of encouragement, let me be quiet while you put the book aside for a few minutes, and explore this meditation for yourself. *Just relax, tune into your breathing, then include your heartbeat/pulse with your breathing, then include your sense of balance, and then experience your whole body at once, here in the present moment:*

3

ANXIETY AND IMMUNE-SYSTEM DYSFUNCTIONS

We all know from experience that falling ill tends to make us feel anxious. Regardless of whether we contract a serious disease or simply get hit with a raging fever for a few hours when we have the flu, any brush with illness reminds us of our own mortality, our own potential to fall so ill we expire.

A basic dimension of sickness is the effect this anxiety has on our recovery systems. Anxiety begins first with the perception that we are sick. Then comes the thinking that projects the sickness into the future and plays with various possibilities, one of them being the development of such an extreme state of sickness that we die.

With this fantasy of possible death comes the emotional reaction of fear. As we will explore step by step in this book, fear is actually a biochemical reaction in the body involving both muscular contractions and glandular secretions that prepare the body to defend itself against danger. If it were possible to fight physically against one's sickness and the danger of death, then the fear reaction would be discharged in action, and there would be no difficulty with this whole process.

But in so many cases, such as illness, there is no physical way to act to deal with the danger. In fact, the danger itself does not exist in the present moment, but is a creation of the future projections of the mind. Thus a chronic state of anxiety is created in the body, a negative condition that adds to the existing state of illness.

Since the 1950s, we have known through research that such anxiety and stress have a negative effect on the functioning of the immune system. Pioneers in this field, such as Robert Adler of the University of Rochester School of Medicine, used classical conditioning to show how animals can be trained to suppress their own immune responses. And numerous studies have demonstrated that animals become increasingly susceptible to infection and disease when subjected to prolonged stress.

More recent research with human beings has shown definitively that emotional conditions such as bereavement following death of a loved one, or serious depression, reduce the ability of the white blood cells (lymphocytes) to react to infection. And in the study of human stress, begun by Hans Selye and refined by research groups throughout the world, there is a definite and deadly link between prolonged anxiety and a progressive dysfunction of the immune system.

But let us put aside the scientific proofs and discussions and turn directly to your present condition to see to what extent anxiety and worry over your condition are creating disturbances in your natural healing process.

To answer this question, we will again want to take a look at your breathing, moment to moment. Anxiety is directly expressed in one's breathing patterns. In fact, anxiety *is* a particular breathing pattern, as I am sure you have noticed from past experiences when you were afraid. Fear generates an instant inhale in the human body, unless the shock of fear is so great that breathing is frozen completely. And in most anxiety reactions, certainly in the case of "illness anxiety," there is a noted imbalance between the inhales and the exhales of a person.

When we are anxious, we seem to be holding our breath on the inhale, or breathing only high in the chest, never exhaling deeply to release the tensions inside us. Pain also generates such an inhale reaction, accompanied by a tensing of the muscles throughout the body.

So for the next few minutes, you might want to take a look at the way you are breathing, and at the muscular tensions in your body, to see if you are holding yourself unconsciously in this anxiety state. In the process, you will find that you can begin to encourage relaxation throughout your body.

RECOVERY SESSION TWO

Whole-Body Stress Reduction

1. First, notice if you feel tension in your chest as you breathe. Take a good, accepting look at your next inhale, your next exhale, and see if your exhale is as deep as your inhale is full. Watch how your breathing changes during your next four to eight breaths.

2. Now turn your attention to your jaw muscles and see if you are holding them tight in an unconscious anxiety stance. Consciously relax your jaw. What about your tongue? As you continue breathing, allow your tongue to relax a little, step by step, breath by breath.

3. Now notice if your throat is constricted, your vocal cords tight, your neck tense. Move your head a little and let the muscles in your neck relax some as you breathe. Breathe through your mouth with an "Ah-h" sound a few times.

4. We now come to the muscles of your shoulders and chest, which directly determine your breathing. Move your shoulders to encourage relaxation, let your breathing deepen as it wants to. And if your physical condition allows, go ahead and stretch a little, even yawn and enjoy a good sigh, to further your relaxation.

5. And what about your belly muscles? Anxiety makes these muscles tense, so that deep abdominal breathing is not even possible. Are your belly muscles habitually held tight? Or conversely, have you let these muscles go completely limp and powerless, with a feeling of hopelessness? Tense them as you exhale; relax them as you inhale.

6. All too often, illness also blocks the free movement of the pelvis, that center of both pleasure and power. In fear, we tense the pelvic muscles and hold this region tight. Pain also generates this contraction. And with prolonged anxiety, where fatigue sets in, the pelvic region totally loses its vitality.
See if you can bring a little vitality into this region by just slightly moving your pelvis as you breathe. When you exhale, contract your stomach muscles and rotate the pelvis up a little in an assertive movement. Then as

you inhale, relax the stomach muscles, arch your back, and let your pelvis move enjoyably down and back slightly.

7. Now notice your legs. Are they tense or relaxed? Try tensing your toes a long moment, then relax them completely. Do the same thing with your fingers. Make a tight fist for a moment as you inhale and hold your breath, then as you exhale, relax your fingers and let a general sensation of relaxation radiate throughout your body.

8. As a final step, you can tense your entire body after an inhale, hold this tension a moment as you hold your breath, and then exhale slowly with a sigh through the mouth, and relax your body completely. This is a basic technique for breaking free of unconscious anxiety tensions in your body, and I would recommend that you do it once an hour, especially if you are lying in bed.

And once you have done this Whole-Body Stress Reduction session, do the Present Moment four-breath meditation. Most probably you will find that you go very deep into your awareness of your body as a whole unified experience.
Breathing / heartbeat / balance / whole body

Such a relaxation recovery session might appear at first glance to be too simple to have any positive effect on your body's ability to heal itself. But recent medical research, such as that done by Allan Goldstein, chairman of the department of biochemistry at the George Washington University School of Medicine, has in fact documented the healing power of effective relaxation techniques.

What Dr. Goldstein found in his research was a statistically significant acceleration in the rate at which lymphocytes in the bloodstream of cancer patients mobilized themselves to attack foreign invaders in the body, when the patient did regular relaxation sessions. This research has been verified in recent studies and stands as a major turning point in our understanding of the relationship between emotional and muscular tensions and reduced immune-system functioning.

So at this point, with what you have learned thus far (the four-word Present Moment meditation, and the Whole-Body Stress Reduction session), you already have an effective program for encouraging your healing process from the inside out. You know that there is scientific verification that this technique works, and without further ado, you are solidly prepared to help your immune system enhance its performance in your healing process.

I encourage you to go back now if you want to, and review these two recovery sessions so that they are successfully memorized and experienced. It is only through taking time away from further reading to learn the exercises step by step that you will gain access to the deeper powers of the programs. Instead of reading through this book as you do other books, as fast as you can, I hope that you will go slowly enough to comprehend fully the different recovery sessions.

4

CELLULAR CONNECTIONS

We have just considered how our minds tend to pull us away from the present moment and into thoughts about the past and the future. In this light, it might appear that thinking is not a mental process that can help in the healing process. But this is not necessarily true, if we know how to approach thinking in a special manner.

Words do have power to affect our bodies. If we think or say a particular word or phrase, we can induce various emotional and physiological reactions in our body, reactions that have been documented quite thoroughly by research.

For instance, when you say the word sex *to yourself, is there any reaction in your body to this word? Try closing your eyes a moment, and say this word three times, on each successive exhale, and see what happens inside you:*

O

If in fact the words we think do affect our bodily functioning, then we must seriously reflect on how we might use this power of the thinking mind to our advantage, rather than to our detriment. If we spend most of our time worrying, which means thinking thoughts that induce anxiety in the body, we are obviously undermining our health. But if we learn to relax our minds and let go of such thoughts (which is exactly what Recovery Sessions One and Two are designed to do), we can break free of at least some of the negative effects our minds have on our health.

In the opposite direction, however, there is much positive benefit to be gained by saying particular words that stimulate a positive flow of emotions through the body. Such words are called *elicitor words*. And for our third recovery session, I want to introduce you to one of the most effective words in the English language for helping in your recovery process.

This word has been around for centuries, and serves as the main label for the internal rebalancing function of the body, which is the central focus of this discussion. The word has been so misused and overused through the years, that at first you might think it has little power at all anymore. But my experience is just the opposite. Once clients open themselves to using this word for Verbal-Cue Activation, they almost always find this third recovery session to be exactly the correct next step in their recovery process.

The word, of course, is *healing*. We could just as easily use the term *immune-system activation*, since it means the same thing. But this new term doesn't have nearly the store of powerful associations in your mind as does *healing*. Whenever you say a word, you stimulate in your mind an awakening of everything you have ever experienced that is associated with that word. And it is this associative power of the mind that makes a single word come alive inside you and evokes a broad range of emotional physiological responses throughout your body.

Curiously, most people who are sick have mixed feelings at first about saying this word and allowing it to resonate throughout their being. Many people who are ill hesitate directly to embrace this word and what it represents. This hesitation reflects the underlying, and usually unconscious, dimension of a personality that is somehow fixated on sickness, thus thwarting the recovery process.

If this is true in your case, please don't be upset. If you regularly turn your attention to the word *healing* and do the following simple meditation on the word, you will find over a period of days that your ability to embrace healing will expand step by step, as long as you don't force it.

RECOVERY SESSION THREE

Verbal-Cue Activation

Recovery Session Three is actually an outgrowth of the first two recovery sessions, and it is best to do them all together, with a slightly different order. Let me talk you through this step by step, so that you have a clear view of the flow of experience I am suggesting.

1. *Begin with the Whole-Body Stress Reduction ses-*

sion you learned in Chapter 3. Give yourself a few min-utes to tune into the tensions in your body, and let them relax.

2. Then go through the four-word Present Moment meditation, so that you bring yourself away from past-future mind trips, and enhance your focus on your physical body in the here-and-now. Notice that we are using four elicitor words in this meditation already, to help focus your attention where you want it: breathing/heartbeat/balance/whole body.

3. And now, as the new step, you will simply add a fifth word, healing, *after you have gone through the first four. On your fifth exhale, say "healing" to yourself. Say the word on your next couple of exhales as well, so that the word sinks in and resonates throughout your consciousness and body awareness. Then just breathe with your mind silent for a few breaths, and open your-self to the unique experience that comes to you, what-ever it may be:*

○

Please don't be jolted if you find that sudden physio-logical sensations rush through your body when you say *healing* to yourself. Such flows of emotional energy are to be encouraged. Many people find that they begin trem-bling during this session, or feel shivers of energy running up and down their spine, or tingling over their skin. The breathing also may change suddenly, as previously blocked energy channels open.

When you feel such emotional changes happening in-side you, open your mouth and breathe freely, so that emotions can be released and healing energy flow more freely. We will talk more about this emotional-release dimension of healing in a later chapter.

I don't want to overprogram you with expectations about this three-phase healing meditation. Each of you will have your own experience; and each time you do the meditation you will have a new experience.

Now, in order to give you the full sequence of events in this healing process, let me now introduce you to Recovery Session Four.

RECOVERY SESSION FOUR

Direct Focusing

Direct Focusing is the technique of turning the mind's attention to the specific region of the body that needs to heal and of holding the mind's attention there for a period of time, usually for between four and twelve full breaths.

Notice what your immediate reaction is, as I suggest that you focus your attention on the injured or diseased part of your body. Watch your breathing and let it speak for you, either with tension of denial and rejection of this suggestion, or with relaxation into what intuitively feels like a worthwhile approach to healing. Don't judge your response or reaction, see it clearly and accept it. Only with this acceptance can you begin to move beyond what may be a negative first feeling.

Many people, especially those with cancer, heart problems, and organ disorders, at first find it almost impossible to focus attention directly, over a period of time, to their diseased region. To look away from what scares you constitutes a natural fear reaction of the system: to ignore a problem in the hope that if you are not aware of it, it may go away. There exists also a widespread—and mistaken—belief that if you focus your attention on an infection, it will only give the infection more energy to expand its brutal dominion in the body.

In any case, the act of turning one's awareness to a diseased region of the body can elicit anxiety and rejection, blocking completely further focusing. If you find that you have this reaction, accept it, and don't force yourself to do this Recovery Session Four program just now.

But if you feel open to the experience, we can continue. *First do all of Recovery Sessions One and Two, bringing your body into a relaxed state, and bringing your mind into full consciousness of your body as a whole. Then, while remaining in this whole-body awareness, turn your attention to the part of your body that needs to heal. Breathe into this special awareness.*

○

Once you have focused your attention on the special region that needs to recover, say the word healing *to yourself while in this expanded state of awareness. And if you want to, place a hand over the region to further the focusing:*

○

A vast possibility of experiences may come to you at this point in the recovery session. You may feel nothing, and simply continue breathing while old thought patterns come to the fore again, taking you away from the recovery session completely. This will happen now and then, and you should just accept it as your present response.

But perhaps you will find that you can indeed hold your attention on both your breathing, your whole body at once, *and* the special region of your body that needs to heal, and as you say the word *healing* to yourself, you may find completely unexpected sensations happening in your body. I do not want to program you about what to expect, because you would then perhaps create fantasies in your mind to simulate what I suggest, thus fooling yourself and avoiding direct experience of your own response. Instead, I will say that you should be open to whatever sensations, emotions, thoughts, and insights that come to you, and just see what happens when you directly elicit the healing state in your body.

I will give you one basic guiding principle: It is essential that you remain aware of your breathing throughout this session. Your breathing is your reality orientation. It is your constant link with your body, keeping you from drifting out of the present moment and into fantasy. And in a special way, as you will discover for yourself, your breathing is the energy pump that sustains your healing attention.

In review: We have now learned a complete immune-system activation program, the first of several. You can do either Recovery Sessions One, Two, and Three as a unit, or One, Two, and Four as a unit.

Recovery Session One: Regaining the Present Moment—a meditation to bring you completely into the experien-

tial moment. The words are breathing, heartbeat, balance, *and* whole body, *one word with each new exhale.*

Recovery Session Two: Whole-Body Stress Reduction—a relaxation technique to break free of anxious breathing and muscle tensions, through focusing on each region of the body and consciously relaxing step by step.

Recovery Session Three: Verbal-Cue Activation—to employ the cue word healing *and induce a general bodily response to the cue word.*

Recovery Session Four: Direct Focusing—to direct consciously the healing energy of the immune system to the region of the body that needs such attention.

In deciding which recovery session series is best for your particular condition, this general rule will help you in your decision:

If you have a general infection affecting your whole body with fever and aches—as in the flu—it is obviously best to do the general, whole-body healing recovery sessions, One, Two, and Three, to stimulate healing throughout your system.

But when your condition is quite specific, such as a cancerous tumor in one region of the body, or a heart condition where a regaining of balance is called for in that region, then Recovery Session Four, Direct Focusing, is usually the best procedure.

The same general logic applies if you suffer from rheumatism and related joint pains. The Whole-Body Stress Reduction session, for instance, will help greatly with overall tensions, and Recovery Session Three will stimulate your basic sense of vitality and health. But it is also recommended to spend at least two sessions a day, perhaps just four to eight breaths, focusing directly

29

on the region of your body that causes specific pain and cramping.

After you have said the word *healing* to yourself, you can also expand the elicitor word into a sentence. You can say "I want to heal myself," for instance, several times, a number of times a day, and allow this thought to move deeply into your being.

I also recommend that you give yourself the freedom, when considering saying "I want to heal myself," to say instead "I don't want to heal myself," if these words come to mind. It is very healthy actually to admit to yourself aloud that there is a certain part of you that resists healing. By saying "I don't want to heal myself," you can get in touch with the negative side of your feelings and attitudes, thus giving them room to express themselves, and letting go of such negative contractions.

Then you can let the positive side of you speak again with "I want to heal myself," or "I am ready to recover from this sickness," or any similar sentence that comes to mind. Play with these verbalizations at least three or four times a day—they can be immensely helpful in attitude growth. Play also with different ways of breathing as you say the sentences to yourself. You can, for instance, inhale as you think "I want," and then exhale on "to heal myself," and do this a number of times, to set up a deep constant chanting power of healing inside you. Try it!

5

EMOTIONS AND THE IMMUNE SYSTEM

There is quite a large body of research completed now that shows how the emotions of anxiety and chronic stress negatively affect the functioning of the immune system. But other emotions are also culprits when it comes to interfering with the natural healing processes of the body. Depression and grief in particular directly inhibit the immune system. People whose long-term mates have just died have a suddenly reduced resistance to disease.

In the other direction, positive emotions such as love, playfulness, contentment, and mastery seem to have a beneficial effect on healing, as demonstrated by Norman Cousins, who literally laughed himself free from the grips of a deadly disease (ankylosing spondylitis).

With this information in mind, many people conclude that if they can just block all bad feelings inside them, they can overcome the dangerous influences of negative emotions. This approach to emotional and physical health unfortunately does not work well, because inhibiting the so-called negative emotions does not make them go away. It simply drives them into more subtle and usually more destructive levels of expression.

What I strongly recommend is just the opposite approach to dealing with your emotions in relation to your health profile. During the last years, my colleagues and I have been developing a process called *Emotional Balancing*, which helps to bring all the emotions into proper relationship with one another. I'll teach you a brief version of this technique, which you can begin to apply to your own emotions.

The key to this Emotional Balancing approach is this: whether or not we like it, we always carry inside us the entire array of emotions that human beings are born with. Emotions are a genetic inheritance—a baby feels an entire assortment of emotions without being taught them. And to the ends of our lives we are in fact walking, talking bundles of many different emotions.

The problem with emotions comes when we learn how to inhibit one or more of them from direct expression. Many people, for instance, block the feeling of anger, turning the emotion back in upon themselves rather than letting the expression go out in a clean discharge toward the person or situation that provoked the emotion. Once the energy of anger is blocked and turned inward, it can cause serious internal health imbalances. Many heart attack patients, for instance, are victims of their inhibited anger, as we will explore in more detail in a later section.

Emotions developed within us because of their survival value. We *need* every single one of the basic dozen emotions with which we are born. And to deny any of them, or overly to accent one of them to the exclusion of others, is to create a serious imbalance within us.

You yourself possess all of the basic emotions. You are capable of responding to different emotionally provocative situations with different feelings and behavior unless those feelings are by habit blocked inside you.

So how would we apply the basic wisdom of homeostasis to the challenge of balancing all our different emotions? Let me teach you the actual Emotional Balancing technique I use with clients, so that you can experience the process for yourself.

RECOVERY SESSION FIVE

Emotional Balancing

This process is based on briefly opening yourself to experience one of the emotions and then letting go of this feeling, so that you can move on to the next.

First see if you can directly wake up the feeling of the particular emotion in the present moment, then let yourself remember or imagine a situation that stimulates this emotion inside you. All of this can happen quite easily within a minute or two.

And then, rather than becoming overly caught in this emotion, let go of it and move on to the next, going fully into this new emotion just as you did with the first one before.

Through this process you can experience all twelve of the basic emotions within twenty minutes to half an hour. And by opening yourself to all the emotions in so short a time, you gain quite a remarkable sense of balance emotionally. You learn how to accept and open yourself to feelings you usually inhibit, and at the same time learn how to let go of these feelings and integrate them with other feelings.

Little children know naturally how to do this basic emotional balancing. Every day in the life of most children, there is ample provocation for them to feel all of the emotions. But children have little ability to block a feeling, and likewise little trouble in letting go of an emotion once the provocation is gone.

As adults, we need to learn how to let our emotions flow as they did when we were younger. I hope you will find the process a liberating experience, as most of my clients do.

Let me list the emotions as I have labeled them for this recovery session, but bear in mind that the labeling is always rather subjective, as there are many different ways in which you can group the basic emotional expressions of human beings. (You might use other words for the same basic emotions, but this list seems fairly comprehensive.) As you read through the list, observe the powerful potential each elicitor word has for stimulating that particular feeling within you. The emotions are: bliss, anger, love, pain, playfulness, fear, passion, grief, hopelessness, mastery, repulsion, peace.

The trick in Emotional Balancing lies in your ability to look at each word as you read it, and to allow the word to stimulate the feelings, memories, and fantasies you carry inside you related to this word. In a moment we will go down the list slowly and deliberately, for a full introduction. Afterward we will run through the list again with the elicitor words only.

As you go through the list, keep in mind the idea of

your relationship with your emotional nature as a whole; we are not simply aiming at an encounter with each separate feeling. The liberating force is tapped only through the integration and interaction of the different emotions within you.

Bliss

I choose bliss as a beginning emotion because I suspect it was our primary feeling while we were in the womb those eternal nine months before we were born. Babies often also experience the bliss state, regularly every day if their living conditions are positive. And if we are lucky, we continue to slip into this blissful state throughout our entire lives.

Bliss is an emotional condition in which we feel no danger, no pain, no hungers—everything is just perfect, and we are able to relax into a pure state of ecstatic contentment. There is a loss of our sense of individuality in the bliss state; we feel one with the universe. Mystics, of course, are the grand celebrators of the bliss state. But their spiritual ecstasies are simply extensions of our everyday moments of pure, unadulterated happiness at being alive and in harmony with our surroundings.

Many people, unfortunately, begin to lose their contact with the bliss state as they grow up. Life becomes a constant state of contraction and tension, anxiety and anger, so that there is simply no time free for opening up and relaxing into the gift of bliss.

I hope that this Emotional Balancing recovery session will help you to open more to the bliss state, because I believe that it is often right in the middle of the bliss state that healing happens. *Relax a moment right now if you want to, and see if you can make contact with this feeling of bliss:*

Anger

See if you can, without effort, say this word to your-self, and then start to feel this feeling in your body.

Where do you feel anger in your body? What muscles contract? Anger is a preparation of the body for defending itself, for being strong enough to protect whatever is in danger. Can you feel this rush of strength into your body as you feel anger?

Many people, of course, have a habit of blocking this very feeling. If as a child you were punished overmuch, and perhaps unfairly, for expressing your personal power and rights, chances are you block this feeling as an adult without even realizing it. If so, you will find this word bothersome to you. When such a negative reaction happens with one of these words, simply observe the reaction inside you, without trying to force anything. Say to yourself, "Hmm, I reject this word, I don't like to even think about anger, let alone feel it in my body. How interesting!"

Conversely, some of you will find that a sudden feeling of anger floods into your body at the very mention of this word. You have the pressure of anger inside you, and perhaps for days, weeks, even years you have been holding in this anger. By not releasing it, of course, you build up quite a backlog of the emotion.

What I recommend, unless you are in a situation where you can really move and shout and release the feeling, is that you breathe into the emotion you feel for a few breaths, and then let go of it and move on to the next word.

Here we have an essential example of emotional balancing: you let yourself feel one emotion, then learn to shift your feelings to another emotion, quite an opposite one, so that you begin to feel freedom from fixation on a particular emotional state.

What you learn from saying the word *anger* and feeling it inside you is that this feeling lives within you, is a part of you, whether or not you are consciously activating it at the time. The feeling, in itself, is neither good nor bad; it is simply one aspect of your overall emotional repertoire. At times when you need strength to protect yourself and your interests, it is invaluable.

Now let us move on to a feeling that lives along with bliss and anger within you.

Love

Breathe and say this word to yourself, and notice how your breathing muscles change their functioning, as you let yourself feel this beautiful feeling in the chest and whole body. See love.

Once you have seen the direct effect of the word on your emotions, on your body, you can see what memories are associated with this word and physical feelings that accompany the memory of moments when you were feeling love toward someone.

Whereas anger is usually felt most in the muscles, love is usually a deeper, internal feeling, related to both breathing and the heart region. Anger tends to tense the jaw muscles; love is a relaxation of these muscles. Similarly, anger tightens the vocal cords, while love relaxes them.

So by going from anger to love, you experience a beautiful "tense-then-release" process that is built into the overall Emotional Balancing.

You will find that you can have anger and love together in your body. We tend to separate our emotions into isolated compartments. But, in fact, we can integrate them, let them be in open relationship with one another, and give each emotion its space inside us, with equal value and respect for its various qualities.

However, the first few times you do this recovery session, please don't expect a total feeling of integration and balance. With all of these sessions, the deeper experiences come through regular practice, as you see what new experiences come each time. Emotional Balancing is something to be done not just once or twice, but throughout one's life.

Pain

Ugh! Who wants to imagine pain? This is something to avoid at all costs, right? Wrong.

Pain is an integral part of life, not something to be denied. If we try to avoid pain, we only give it undue emphasis through this very denial. It is best to allow pain its own equal place in the parade of emotions, rather than shutting it out of mind when possible.

I know that some of you are currently suffering from serious pain as you read this, and I hope that you can direct your open attention to this feeling for a few breaths, and then experience shifting your attention to the next emotion. This will help develop a freedom to move from pain to other feelings, rather than a fixation on the pain you feel. What I am offering, basically, is an escape route. But it first requires direct experience of the pain before shifting to other possible emotional states.

Experience your pain now, and if you are not in pain, still allow yourself to remember what it feels like to hurt. There is a tensing of the muscles, as in anger, and a general contraction away from the point of pain. With pain, you tend to inhale and hold your breath. What other muscular reactions do you feel when you experience pain in your body? And what memories come to you of past painful experiences?

By regularly opening yourself to the reliving of painful experiences in the past, you can free yourself from the unconscious tensions that may be held in your body as a habit. People carry with them for years, even for a lifetime, tensions that developed during times of extreme pain and suffering. Through this technique, you can begin to free yourself from habitual contractions that only undermine your health.

The basic experience with this word is this: yes, I know pain, I have hurt badly in the past, perhaps even now. And I can let go of this pain!

Let go by saying this opposite word to yourself as you read it now:

Playfulness

By playfulness I mean that childhood freedom to lose yourself totally in having fun—to be completely immersed in a beautiful world of your own creation, where nothing exists in the moment but this playful state.

Playfulness is a feeling in the body, in the muscles, a feeling of power and relaxed pleasure together in the present moment, with no thought of past or future. Play is, in essence, a present-moment experience with no conflict or pain.

So let yourself feel this feeling in your arms, your heart, your whole body at once, and then see what memories come to mind of times when you were in a playful state. Let your breathing be your guide, and perhaps close your eyes.

Fear

Fear is an emotion that most of us wish we had never been born with. Fear is not fun at all. It is a shock to the system and, when prolonged into a chronic state of anxiety, is extremely painful in its own particular way, in terms of muscular tensions and inner contractions that generate mental suffering as well.

But is fear really this terrible emotion that does us nothing but harm?

What is fear, actually? It is a contraction in the body, a sharp inhalation of breath to fill the lungs with oxygen, and an instant array of glandular secretions that send adrenaline throughout the system, generating, in an instant, a total readiness of the body for action.

All of our emotions developed because of their survival value, over millions of years. Fear stands at the top of the list in terms of survival value—or at least it did in the old days when most of our fears were caused by dangers to our physical well-being.

Fear takes us from a relaxed state to a powerful, charged state, one in which we are ready to fight or to run from danger. Without this reflex of fear, we would have no chance of, say, jumping out of the way of an unexpected car.

The problem with fear is that as human beings, we can generate this state in our bodies simply by imagining a danger that might come in the future, or by remembering a danger we experienced in the past. Only as long as our fear is a response to the present moment is it to our advantage to have this emotion.

It may be a generalization, but human beings these days tend to be quite full of the kind of fear that is past and future oriented. We have a habit of keeping ourselves overwhelmed, through the news media, with bad and scary things that have happened all over the world each day; and then the chronic pattern of worrying about which of these bad things might happen to us in the future.

So take this step in Emotional Balancing: feel the anxiety in your body intensely for a few breaths; become really conscious of the fear inside you, letting memories of fear experiences rise to the surface; then move on to the next word.

Passion

Just as we are all born with the ability to feel fear, we are also born with the opposite ability, that of feeling extreme positive charging in the body, especially when we find ourselves in arousing situations where the full response of sexual desire is elicited.

Even if you are sick, let yourself feel this passion in your body for a few breaths. Feel it change your breathing, for instance, as you see the word. Say it to yourself so it vibrates throughout your body.

Passion is a mixture of compassion and power. Whereas compassion can be a quiet, passive experience, passion itself is active, pushed by a most beautiful hunger toward satisfaction and fulfillment. (Passion is not only sexual hunger, it can be a hunger for anything. We have a passion for great music, a lust for wild snow-swept walks, a hunger for superb cooking and wines, and so on.)

Let yourself remember times when you were full of passion, remember the feeling in your body, relive the experience that comes to you.

Grief

People die and leave us alone in life, or people we love and are attached to leave us and break our hearts with feelings similar to those we might have had they died. Grief is a universal human experience. Are you open to feeling it for a few breaths, to experience this emotion inside you?

Remember that if you do not open yourself to one or more of these words it is perfectly all right for now. Everyone tends to block and avoid certain emotions, while being overly fixated on others. Through this recovery session, you are finding out which emotions you try to escape from habitually and which ones you feel quite freely. Each time you do this recovery session, you will have a new experience. There will be plenty of time for new openings to come to you, step by step.

Grief that is not released, not fully experienced, can be a major cause of illness. Studies have shown that the immune-system functioning of people who have lost a mate is seriously reduced during the months of bereavement. This direct relationship between grief and reduced immune-system functioning should be expanded to include people suffering from broken hearts as well as from the death of a loved one.

Grief is actually a mixture of different feelings, which, when put together, feel like grief, abandonment. There is an empty hopeless feeling, first, as if our own self has been somehow lost. And right in the middle of this feeling is the sudden anger of a three-year-old who is angry at being left alone. And somewhere in the midst of abandonment and anger, there is acceptance and a fighting spirit to rise again and go on with life.

Open yourself to the feeling of grief for a few breaths; let it be there, and see what memories come to mind.

Hopelessness

For all of us, life sometimes feels hopeless. Many people, when sick, try to pretend that this feeling never comes to them. But of course, with serious illnesses especially, the feeling of hopelessness is sure to appear sometimes. If you push it away, it will simply work at unconscious levels to undermine your health. You do better to give this emotion its space of a few breaths, to remember times when you were caught in the past by total despair. *See what comes to you now as you experience for a moment the despair that comes when life seems hopeless, when you just want to give up and die. Breathe into it.*

Mastery

We tend to overlook this emotion, but for a balanced emotional condition, the feeling of mastery, of being able to do something in life well, is essential. Even if a small ability, it should be counted. Human beings need this emotion in order to sustain their lives. All too often we are blocked in letting ourselves feel pride in our accomplishments, in our abilities, in our mastery of chosen areas of expertise.

Let yourself feel the emotion of successful performance. This is a wonderful feeling, especially in the chest. See what memories come to mind, of things you have done in the past in a masterly way.

Very often, sick people are caught in a feeling of helplessness, of uselessness. If this is your case, you can do something directly, now, to regain your feeling of potency. It doesn't matter what it is you do well; just exercise your ability to perform some work in a masterly manner. If you can hardly move in your present condition, do things with your mind. Practice visualization, for instance, until you perfectly visualize a friend's face. Or develop your mastery over memory by remembering the words to a song or the theme of a symphony.

However, we want to keep this emotion in balance with the rest, and so we move on to the final two in our twelve:

Repulsion

Along with feelings of love and excitement, we have inside us an opposing feeling of repulsion, a feeling stimulated by any situation that somehow violates our self-esteem, or that more directly threatens our integrity, physically or emotionally. We can be repulsed by the sight of blood, by the smell of dead bodies, by the thought of liver frying in a pan, by the face of some person, by the atmosphere in a particular room.

So go ahead and let yourself breathe into a few moments of this feeling. See also what memories come to mind, of times when you were overcome with the feeling of repulsion.

Peace

Finally, to round off the full array of human emotions, we have a special feeling that comes to us when everything is relaxed in our lives, at least for a moment, when we are satisfied, when we need not push to survive right now, when all our hungers are taken care of and we can pause and feel peace.

Babies who are treated even reasonably well know the state of peace intimately. Little children experience this emotional condition regularly. But all too often, as we grow older, we let anxieties and pressures dominate our emotional lives, so that peace doesn't get its fair room to exist inside us.

Say the word peace *as you read it, take it inside you, and see what happens. See what feelings come into your body, and also what memories come to the surface, memories of times when you were in a state of peace, perhaps lying in the sun, or floating in the ocean, or lying in your lover's arms after making love—see what your own experiences have been, and feel your own po-*

tential for feeling this way now, even in the midst of an
illness or injury. Peace.

○

The Twelve Emotions at a Glance

Bliss
Anger
Love
Pain
Playfulness
Fear
Passion
Grief
Hopelessness
Mastery
Repulsion
Peace

Your basic personality is rooted in the way you express or
inhibit the flow of emotions through your body. Emotions
are not abstract concepts. They are physical happenings
inside your body. This is why they affect your immune
system so strongly. The healthy body is one that regularly
experiences all emotions in proper balance in response to
events around the body and to inner thoughts and fantasies.

People who are sick are almost always inhibiting certain feelings, partly through old habit and partly through
the provocation of the illness. They are also almost always
stuck in one or two emotions during the sickness, emotions
that are usually detrimental to the recovery process. As

you went down the list above, you may have noticed which emotions were hard for you to relate to and experience and which ones seemed to reflect your chronic state. These differences show you where you are out of balance emotionally; by regularly repeating the Emotional Balancing recovery session you can bring yourself back into balance again.

Now, below, I repeat the elicitor words. It is best not to linger on any one emotion. As you go down the concise outline below look at each word for a few breaths; close your eyes and see what feelings, memories, come to you. Then, after no more than two or three minutes, open your eyes, come into the present moment again, take a deep breath, and look at the next word. It is this moving from one emotion to the next that is the key.

1. BLISS *(happiness, joy)*
      feel pure joy in your body
      remember times of ultimate bliss
      imagine an experience of perfect happiness

2. ANGER *(frustration, aggression)*
      feel anger in your muscles
      remember exploding with anger
      imagine venting your aggressions

3. LOVE *(acceptance, compassion)*
      let your heart expand in love
      remember being deeply in love
      imagine a beautiful loving experience

4. PAIN *(suffering, contraction)*
      feel pain in your body
      remember terrible times of suffering
      imagine the most horrible pain

5. PLAYFULNESS *(spontaneous fun)*
      feel playful in your body

remember playing when you were young
imagine a playful fantasy

6. FEAR *(anxiety, apprehension)*
    feel the contractions of fear
    remember times of intense anxiety
    imagine being scared

7. PASSION *(desire, lust, hunger)*
    feel the beautiful rush of desire in your body
    remember wild, lustful experiences of your
        past
    let your fantasy conjure up ultimate moments
        of passion

8. GRIEF *(mourning, heartbreak)*
    open yourself to the feelings of grief
    remember times of terrible heartbreak
    imagine ultimate grief

9. HOPELESSNESS *(depression, despair)*
    let total depression overcome you
    remember times of terrible depression
    imagine being completely hopeless

10. MASTERY *(pride, achievement)*
    feel pride in who you are
    remember doing something extremely well
    imagine being a master at something special

11. REPULSION *(rejection, nausea)*
    feel nausea in your throat and stomach
    remember times of ultimate repulsion and
        nausea
    imagine the ultimately nauseating situation

12. PEACE *(contentment, satisfaction)*
    relax into quiet satisfaction and peace

remember times of complete contentment
imagine the ideal peaceful experience

You now have a simple method for waking up all twelve of the emotions within you, without indulging in any one of them, or getting stuck in any of them that you don't like overmuch. I hope that my brief introduction to this deep balancing process has been clear enough so that you can now use this basic list as a regular healing session. Devote a half hour at least twice a week, if you are ill.

6

NEUROLOGICAL CONNECTIONS

Research over thousands of years has shown that there are different energy centers in the body, primarily at special locations along the spinal column. Ancient yoga masters charted these centers quite precisely, and developed complex and powerful means of activating these centers through yoga postures and breathing meditations.

From a very different perspective, Wilhelm Reich explored the different emotional energy centers of the human body and, perhaps not surprisingly, placed the emotional centers in the same basic locations in the body.

Among the Guatemalan Indian traditions that I studied a number of years ago while doing fieldwork in that region is an ancient Mayan one that locates eight primary energy centers in the human body, supposedly centers where the various gods could communicate with the more highly advanced members of Mayan society.

And fairly early in the neurological exploration of the human nervous system by modern science, concentrated groupings of nerve fibers were found in precisely the locations along the spine where the three previously described traditions had located them.

For as many as three thousand years, the Tantric yoga practitioners of Tibet and northern India have advanced the techniques for balancing these various centers of the body through quite a complicated and difficult movement and meditation procedure. This technique consciously opens centers where the flow of energy is blocked, and reduces the flow where too great an accumulation of energy has developed.

When I speak of energy in this regard, I am not talking about an esoteric imaginary flow of mystic power through the body, but refer rather to easily measurable electric pathways that exist throughout the body, along the meridian lines that have been used for countless years by the practitioners of acupuncture.

Wilhelm Reich was among the first doctors to measure the increased energy flow over the surface of the skin during different emotional-discharge states. Our emotions powerfully alter the energy state of the body in general. In addition, a person often can block the flow of energy through one or more centers in the body, such as the heart, the pelvis, the eyes, the throat. The blocking appears to be an integral aspect of disease development in these regions.

What is critical here is not gross energy flow, but the balancing of this energy flow through all different centers of the body. How do we bring about a successful energy balance throughout the body, with techniques that are practical for the average person?

A number of years ago, a research team at Duke University performed an extremely significant experiment. They tested a faith healer, who supposedly had the power to heal people by placing his hands on the diseased parts of their body. This "laying on of hands" tradition has been popular in various Christian sects for the entire duration of the Christian religion, but medical understanding of the physical functioning of the body ran directly counter to any such possibility.

An ingenious experimental technique was designed, to prove once and for all that there is no such thing as a healing power of human hands. The outcome of the research was anticipated to be, obviously enough, negative. A particular bacterial culture was known to die at a certain rate over a certain period of time, and the challenge to the healer was to use his hands to keep the bacteria alive.

Simply put, he did.

Our hands are intimately connected with a considerable part of the brain's total volume. We use our hands for major aspects of our survival, both for physical manipulation of the outside world and for sensory relating with objects around us. If we want to focus the mind's attention to a particular part of the body, we can do this most effectively by placing the hand over that part of the body.

I am not, however, asking you to believe that your hands have healing power. We do not need a belief, one way or the other, for this particular technique to be useful. What I recommend instead is that you approach this recovery session with an open mind; see what you experience directly in using your hands to bring about an integration of your energy centers; and then direct healing attention where needed at the time.

In the Mayan tradition, at least among the particular highland Guatemalan tribe that I studied, the hands are placed over two energy centers at the same time, to encourage a communication and a harmony between the two gods who supposedly underlie the chosen centers. The ancient tradition held that illness in a person meant a war was going on between two or more centers (gods) and that placing hands over these centers and breathing in a particular way could induce the gods to make peace with each other.

We needn't concern ourselves with the religious aspect of this technique; the use of hands in this manner seems to work powerfully without any particular belief system. There are certainly underlying spiritual dimensions to life, if by spiritual we mean all those vast realms in life and death that science cannot touch. But my observation has been that successful healing does not presuppose complex belief systems. I always advise clients to open themselves to whatever spiritual healing energy they may find, but at the same time take responsibility themselves for bringing about balance in their nervous system, emotions, thoughts, and muscular system.

So let us focus on your own hands, as they are, without metaphysical projections, and see what you experience as you place these hands over your energy centers in a particular way that encourages integration of the centers.

To begin, however, we need to review briefly the various centers that have been found in the human body. For my purposes I have combined yoga *chakras,* bioenergetic centers, and the neurological centers into one holistic system and taken the freedom of adding one extra center that is usually ignored in the various traditions.

Sexual Center

There is no doubt but that human beings have the potential for increasing or reducing the energy potential of this first center of the body. I prefer to think of this center, in fact, as the creation center, for it is the energy point where the actual creation of new beings happens in the body.

All too often, during childhood, children develop difficulties in integrating this center into the other centers, and the resulting energy imbalance tends to distort the entire emotional and physiological functioning of the person. Learning to integrate the sexual center into the other centers is of utmost importance.

Each of these centers has a special location in the body, and I suspect that you can already guess where this center is found.

Power Center

The human body has its center of equilibrium and also its center of personal power directly above the genitals, just below the belly button. This center is called the *"ki energy"* center in Oriental martial arts traditions. And in the emotional tradition of Wilhelm Reich also, this is where a person's main power energy emanates from. If you want to feel this for yourself, push against a wall and notice where your focus of attention is centered while pushing. You can just imagine pushing a car, and feel this also.

Once again, childhood training often disturbs our relationship with our power center. Either we tend to be overactive in this center or, conversely, we tend to block the center, to reduce our power so as not to provoke punishment. To integrate our feeling of power into our other centers will be vital for balancing success. We can see already that a person's sexual expression and his or her personal power expression often come together. And as a first step in the Hand-Directed Integration recovery session, you will place one hand over your sexual center, the other over your power center. I will describe the actual process to you once we have reviewed the various centers.

Breathing Center

This center is found in the solar plexus, that spot just below the front of your rib cage where, if someone hits you there, you get the air knocked out of you. Your stomach and several vital organs are located in this region as well; an integration of this center into the others is a direct path to overall balance in the system.

Heart Center

Along with the breathing reflex, the constant beating of your heart is, as we saw earlier, your main life-support mechanism. To place your hands over these two centers at once is a beautiful feeling. Often, the emotional experiences associated with the heart region are very powerful, and quite often either too much or too little energy is fixated in this region. We speak of a cold heart, a broken heart, a bleeding heart. When the energy flow here is out of balance for a period of time, health problems are likely to occur.

I would suggest that when you place a hand over this region, you put it over the center of the chest, rather than over the heart itself, because the actual energy center, related to nerve groupings in the spine, is centered over the spine, not the heart.

Throat Center

We all know how emotions become constricted in the throat region. Our thyroid gland is located here, as well as our means of vocalization, the vocal cords. This is also especially where blockage of the flow of energy between the head and the body is concentrated. An imbalance here is both painful emotionally and dangerous to your health. You will often have your strongest experiences when you have a hand over your heart and one over your throat. Your breathing, of course, is also controlled by this narrow passageway from lungs to mouth.

Mouth Center

This center is not mentioned in the yoga tradition, but I list it because it plays such a vital role in emotional expression, and is such a strong locale for the blocking of energy in the body. Along with the mouth, it includes the jaw and tongue muscles, which tense when there is an imbalance of energy in this region. Chronic tight jaws are a certain indicator of energy imbalance and of health complications to follow.

Eye Center

As I have written in depth in other publications (see Bibliography), our eyes are a primary center of the body, determining much of our contact with the outer world. They also reveal much of our inner feelings, when we allow these feelings to flow out of the eyes and be seen by others.

But we tend to inhibit the flow of this emotional expression out of the eyes if we are punished by this "doorway to our souls"; and when we block the energy flow in this region, our entire balance is thrown off. So placing your hand over your eyes, while you have the other hand over your mouth, will almost always lead to a deep experience.

Brain Center

We now come to that region or energy center of the body that is so profusely active with neurochemical flows. Our brain is, of course, central headquarters for the whole performance of the body.

When you place a hand over your forehead region, you are directing your mind to itself. Usually, when you place your hand over your forehead, you will notice a quieting of your thoughts.

With one hand over your eyes, and the other over your forehead, you are bringing seeing (internal as well as external) into harmony with thinking. I do not want to go into an intellectual discussion about this balancing position; you should have your own experiences, free of my suggestions. I will say only that once your mind is quiet, there will still be a quiet activity. It is important to get in touch with this quiet activity.

Crown Chakra

I use this term from the yoga tradition for the last energy center. For yoga masters, the crown chakra was the highest center; the sexual chakra, the absolute lowest. For Wilhelm Reich and enthusiasts of emotional discharge, however, the sexual center was considered the highest; the crown chakra was simply the place where you put your hat! For me, a combination of both attitudes seems best.

The crown chakra is the top of your head. When you put your hand over this center, you will have completed the exploration of the nine energy centers with which we are going to work.

You now have an overview of the different centers in your body. I'm sure you can already see that we are going to approach these centers with much the same spirit that we approached the balancing of the various emotions in Recovery Session Five. In fact, you will notice that each physical center tends to be highlighted by the emotional feelings experienced in that region of the body.

RECOVERY SESSION SIX

Hand-Directed Integration

This recovery session can be done either standing up, sitting down, or lying on your back. If possible, I recommend that you try it in all three positions, because each position yields quite a different experience.

Most often, people do this Hand-Directed Integration recovery session lying down. You can do it quickly, in a few minutes, or you can take up to half an hour to do it. Once you have gone through the Hand-Directed Integration procedure, I suggest a short healing session employing the Direct Focusing technique already learned, and, further, if you are interested, another American Indian healing approach called Earth Focus, which we will learn later on.

For now, let me guide you through the Hand Integration. You will want to practice the simple progression of hand positions a few times to memorize the movements, before going deeply into the experience itself.

First, make yourself comfortable, lying or sitting where you won't be disturbed for a period of time (although disturbance isn't a serious problem with this session; you can always start over if disturbed).

PHASE 1. *Relax. Watch your breathing without making any effort to control it. Let your breathing stop when it wants to, and start up without effort, so that you feel directly the breath reflex that sustains your breathing.*

PHASE 2.   *When the word comes naturally to you, say* breathing *to yourself as you exhale. Then inhale with a quiet mind, and on your second exhale, say* heartbeat, *and see if you can feel your pulse somewhere in your body. Inhale quietly, then on the third exhale, say* balance *to yourself, and move your body so you feel your muscles and bones in relationship to gravity. Inhale, and on your fourth exhale, say* whole body, *and experience this expanded state of awareness that you learned in Recovery Session One.*

PHASE 3.   *We now come to the Hand Integration session itself. First, focus your attention on your two hands as you observe your breathing for three or four breaths. Tune into the brain/hands contact.*

1. *Now place one of your hands on the* sexual/creation *center, and say this word to yourself. Without trying to make anything happen in your awareness, simply focus on this hand on this center for a few breaths.*

2. *Then place your other hand on your* power *center, and say the word* power *to yourself as you exhale. Say the word slowly, and so that you feel it in the muscles of your throat. In the same way that we used verbal cue words to elicit emotional feelings, we are now using verbal cues to awaken everything associated with this power center of your body. But please don't think that I mean you to start "thinking about" power at this point. Quite the contrary: I expect that, by saying this word slowly to yourself as you exhale, you will quiet your mind of intellectual activity and turn your attention to the pure experience coming to you.*
You now have one hand on your sexual/creation center, and the other hand on the power center. You might want to say to yourself at this point, "Creativity

and power, together" and see how these words evoke adeeper experience.

3. *When you feel ready, move your lower hand up to the* breathing *center, so that you have one hand on the power center and one on the breathing center. Say* breathing *to yourself, and see what experiences come to you. Each time you will have a different experience. I have done this recovery session hundreds of times and never become bored—on the contrary, our consciousness regularly expands through such a meditative process, so that we are always discovering new realms of balance and interaction between the various centers.*

When you are ready, you can say, "Power and breathing, together."

4. *And then when you want to, move your lower hand up to your* heart *center, and integrate heart and breathing in like manner as you have the first centers.*

You have now brought all the four centers of the lower part of your body into a new harmony and relationship. If you want, you can reverse the process and go back downward, to further this process.

5. *Now bring the lower hand up and place it on your* throat, *that connection between the lower body and the head. As before, say* throat *to yourself further to focus your attention on this region. Breathe a few times and see what you experience under your hands. Usually, the muscles of the throat will relax at this point, and breathing will deepen. Saying "Heart and throat, together," also deepens the experience.*

6. *When you are ready, move the lower hand up to your* mouth, *and repeat the process as before. Let your*

jaw muscles relax, and your tongue also, and feel the connection all the way up your body, from the creation center, through the power center, into the breathing center, on up to the heart center, then upward through the throat, to the mouth, so that you can feel directly this total connection from bottom to top—another expanding experience related to being aware of your whole body at once.

7. *And when you want to, move your lower hand up to your* eyes, *and repeat the process as before. Your eyes will be encouraged to relax through this attention. In fact, you will notice, as we have shown in research, that when you place your hand on a region of your body, that region does tend to relax—a basic fact to remember.*

8. *Now bring your lower hand up and place it on your* forehead, *saying* mind *to yourself. This posture will almost certainly feel quite good to you, and you want to be sure to remain aware of your breathing to allow your consciousness to expand as it wants to.*
Sometimes your arms will become tired while holding these postures. Be sure to relax your shoulders as much as possible and always feel free to put your arms and hands down for a while when you need to. There is no problem in breaking the flow of this exercise, so feel free to do it just as you wish, once you have learned the basic structure.

9. *And now, bring your lower hand up and place it on the* top of your head. *This is another position that feels quite wonderful for most people, with the two hands in this posture.*

10. *When you are ready, you can move your lower hand down to the creation/sexual center, so that you*

focus your attention on your entire nervous system at once, between the two hands. Breathe into whatever experience comes.

And then put your hands down at your sides when you want to, and relax completely, holding your breathing as your center, and see what experience comes to you at this point.

You have now done the basic Hand-Directed Integration session for your different energy centers. I will not program you with expectations of what often happens with other people in this recovery session. I want to leave you completely free to have a unique experience each time you do it. We must be careful that we don't fall victim to hypnotic suggestion in this sort of healing work. I could tell you what might happen to you when you do this exercise, and then your mind would conjure up a fantasy of the experience I described, and you would have such a fantasy and even think that it was a direct personal experience, forgetting that I had just programmed your fantasy with the idea.

Similarly, be careful of the following mind game that often limits the newness of such recovery sessions: once you do this exercise and have a powerful experience—perhaps on the first time, but most likely on the fourth or fifth time you do it—you will be tempted to expect the same powerful experience the next time you do the session. And if you are not careful, you will start to create a similar experience in your fantasy, combining memory with direct experience, so that you lose the newness of the session. Please remember this: never anticipate having the same experience twice. You will never, ever truly repeat the same experience, with this or any other activity.

If, during any of these recovery sessions, you find yourself bored, having the same experience over and over again, then you know that you have lost your direct contact with the present moment, and are caught in expectations and fantasies of what has happened to you in the past.

To break free of this, first, never force yourself to do any of the sessions. Do them only when you want to, and do them because you are eager to explore your healing potential, not because you want to force healing on yourself. Second, put special emphasis on remaining aware of your breathing, moment to moment, so that your whole-body experience is heightened.

○

Healing Hands

As you relax, focus on your hands again and say the word healing *to yourself a couple of times. Just see how this word resonates in your system. Notice particularly if you do feel healing energy in your hands at this point. If not, fine. But if there is some energy available, you can breathe without effort, and let your hands move on their own, and go anywhere on your body that they want to, wherever healing energy and attention is needed at the moment. And say* healing *when you want to, to enhance the process.*

This is a very simple but very deep experience, and I encourage you to do it without any of the heaviness that people often associate with the "laying on of hands." Don't expect anything to happen; just let your hands rest where they want to, and stay with your breathing, saying the word *healing* when you want to.

Let your hands keep moving where they want to go, and let them massage any part of your body that they want to. You will need little instruction for this, because you will find it to be a natural process.

Let your hands go to areas that need healing attention not only in terms of physical pain and difficulty but also emotional pains and contractions. If you like, you can say, "I want to heal myself," or a similar sentence, to enhance the power of the session. And if you have been lying on your back, whenever you want to end the session, roll over onto your stomach, and just rest and reflect for a while.

As a more structured approach to this recovery session, you can explore what you experience when you place your hands on different pairs of centers, so that you consciously bring together usually separate energy centers. For instance, place one hand on the heart and the other on the power center to bring these two together.

Try all the different combinations possible over the next few weeks. One hand on the forehead/mind, the other on the heart, is another example of a powerful combination. Experiment for yourself and see what integration you generate.

By the way, you do not have to go through the entire nine-center integration process in each recovery session. Very often, people go halfway through the process, then find that their hands do not want to move on, that there is a special feeling under the hands where they are; for instance, when the hands are on the heart and the throat. Perhaps, then, you should remain in this position for the rest of the session. Go ahead and make the process suit your particular inclinations at the time.

Emotional Healing

Often, while people are practicing the Hand-Directed Integration and healing session, unexpected emotional pressures begin to build in the body, pressures stimulated by the session itself. Feeling emotional pressure inside is a positive development if you open yourself to the emotion and let it come out.

Of course, you may have to limit your emotional release depending on your physical condition at the time, and on consideration of people who may be around you. But let me give you a general, if challenging, suggestion: rank yourself and your emotional expression as the most important elements in your life, more important than the upsetting of people who themselves may have inhibitions about emotional expression, and who may be afraid of your emotional releases. Your main responsibility is to allow your healing process to be activated. It is counterproductive to be more worried about what people will think about your behavior than to give yourself the freedom to release emotions that might be central in your illness. I say this emphatically here, because I have known too many people who actually withered and died of a disease rather than break free of their friends' restrictions on the expression of forbidden emotions. Chronic inhibition of emotional flow in the body, especially the flows of anger and sorrow, is a primary factor in the development of disease. Allowing yourself the freedom to let your emotions out can be essential to turning a positive corner in your recovery process.

It is quite common for people who are sick to find themselves feeling strong emotions that were habitually blocked in normal life. Illness is beautiful in this way, in that it stops you, breaks you out of your normal habits, and provides the time and space for you to indulge in feelings that have for too long been inhibited.

But people taking care of you are usually frightened

when a sick person, for instance, starts crying. They will do everything to make you stop your emotional release rather than give you space to release the emotions that are perhaps poisoning you inside. If this is a problem, I recommend that you discuss it with people around you. Tell them that it is healthy for you to release your feelings, and that you want the freedom to do so.

We now come to the question of whether you give *yourself* permission to release your feelings, to express your inside pressures to the outside world. Many people would rather die than let someone catch them crying. Men are especially notorious for this prohibition of an expression of "weakness." Women, on the other hand, often inhibit their expression of anger, fearing to let the outside world see the powerful rage that is sometimes inside. Immune-system dysfunction can be a result of such blocking.

The Emotional Balancing recovery session already learned is, of course, one necessary dimension to this question of emotional health. But you might find, after doing that session, that one of those twelve emotions is under pressure inside you. What do you do?

RECOVERY SESSION SEVEN

Emotional Release

The basic procedure is this: whenever you find yourself with emotional pressure inside you, whether you are swallowing tears or clenching your jaw against the expression of anger, if possible, stop whatever you are doing, and lie on your back, breathe through the mouth. The simple act of breathing through the mouth deeply for a period of time is the main vehicle for allowing emotions to come out and be gone.

It is best to have your knees bent and your feet flat on the floor or bed for this, but it is not essential. What is important is putting yourself in this position for optimum, and safe, release of your feelings.

In this position, you can cry like a baby if you want. And very often, in the middle of the crying comes sudden anger. Pound with your hands and arms, pound the floor with your feet—you won't damage anything. Quite the reverse: you will experience a beautiful release of buried feelings that have probably been contracting your body for years.

Be sure to ask yourself this question: What is more important, not upsetting people around you with emotional release sounds, or recovering from your illness?

You will, of course, have to moderate this recovery session to match your health condition at the moment. I am offering a basic format for emotional release, and you can alter this however you need to, even if you find you must let your tears or anger flow only when completely alone at night. How you do this is secondary. What is vital is letting it happen. You have a right to your feelings, after all. Past conditioning that inhibited your emotions must ultimately be put aside so that you regain emotional balance and have maximum chance of recovering from your illness.

The release of emotions almost always feels good in itself. Genuine anger is a most beautiful rush of feelings, and the discharge through movement and vocalization is a fine feeling!

The negative side of emotional release is the fear you feel in expressing your emotions. Many of us were punished so severely, if sometimes subtly, as children, for expressing forbidden emotions that we have a deathly fear of letting these same emotions come out, even as adults. So I know that for many of you, releasing the feelings that come up will at first be frightening and seem impossible.

Go easy with yourself. Notice what emotions you do feel inside. Watch your blocking habits a number of times. And little by little, begin to accept these forbidden feelings inside you. Even make friends with them secretly. Remember yourself as a two-year-old, with the wild free expression of your feelings. Let that early spirit come back inside you. That spirit, as we shall see later in our Memory Balancing session, can have a most powerful effect on your ability to recover your good health.

I also recommend that you find someone you can really talk with about your feelings, about what you are experiencing day to day. For such a relationship to work, of course, you will need to do an equal amount of listening. Talking is perhaps our main vehicle for emotional expression. If you don't have anyone to talk with right now, talk to yourself, express your deeper feelings at least inwardly, so that you become more emotionally honest with yourself. And be sure to look for the humorous, as well as the serious!

7

PROPER FOODS FOR RECOVERY

The substances that we take into our bodies regularly will obviously determine the general vitality of our bodies. Chronic overeating and the habitual intake of unhealthy foods are two main ingredients in the development of poor health. And when you are ill, the question of food intake is especially crucial.

What do animals, through the wisdom of their instincts, do when they fall ill? Do they continue to eat regularly, eat more, eat less? In almost all cases, they stop eating almost completely when sick. This natural fasting response to illness serves the purpose of giving the digestive system a rest, so that internal balancing processes can operate at maximum efficiency.

Many nutrition experts believe that we should fast one day a week, throughout our lives, in order to give our system a regular chance to cleanse itself of impurities and to burn the excess fats that have accumulated.

The traditions in which health seems optimal, and life span the longest, have this regular fasting as a cultural imperative.

For most of us, however, the idea of going without food for even twenty-four hours seems impossible. Our conditioned hungers become so insistent when we miss even one meal that to think of going without food for a day, seven days, or a month is impossible.

In truth, though, we can do very well without any food intake for quite a few days. Substantial research has proved such fasting does not hurt our bodies, but indeed it accomplishes the opposite: fasting cleanses the body of toxins that have been stored in fatty tissue, the liver, and other organs. It also purifies the blood, tones the organs, and balances the digestive system for optimum functioning.

Besides this physiological help, fasting helps balance the emotions and thought habits, breaking us free of habitual patterns and completely shifting energy flows in the body. Almost all spiritual traditions include regular fasting as part of the process of spiritual purification and growth.

I give such loud praise to fasting because, for many ill people, it can be the turning point in their recovery experience. So consider fasting one day a week, if this meets with your doctor's approval. Or you can simply give up breakfast and begin your eating day with lunch, so that your body has all night and all morning for the purification process. If you want to explore a longer fast, you should speak with your doctor, and also to a nutrition expert who teaches fasting, in order to proceed correctly. For many ill people, a fast of one week or even ten days, when done under supervision, can have remarkable healing results. Your entire personality will have the chance to go through a transformation, and your life habits as well. I emphasize the need for proper supervision in undertaking such a fast; I also recommend that you read books on the topic.

But for most of us simple changes in diet can also effect positive immune-system functioning. I will give you some guidelines to consider in your own diet.

A general rule, during sick periods of your life, is to avoid foods heavy in animal fat. If you have a habit of eating meat regularly, even when sick, see if you can put this aside for the time being, as much as possible. The same goes for eggs. Also, reduce dairy foods such as milk and cheese to a minimum, especially if you are in bed and not exercising much. Such animal-fat foods will further clog up your system.

However, I do not believe in forcing a sick person to give up pleasurable eating completely. Now and then indulge in whatever you like, so that your pleasure in eating is not lost.

But you will find, especially when you are sick, that very simple foods will begin to taste very good to you, and that smaller helpings will suit you better than large ones. Take breakfast. Ham and eggs, or bread and cheese, can be put aside in exchange for what is considered an optimal breakfast by nutrition experts.

The Perfect Breakfast

The basic principle behind this breakfast recipe, and in fact the entire dietary advice in this chapter, is that you eat foods that are full of their own life, rather than dead foods. By dead foods, we mean dead animal flesh, for instance, especially processed meats. Canned vegetables are equally "dead," overcooked and preserved. Wheat flour itself is a far cry from its more vital form, a whole, potent seed with the life-force intact.

Seeds themselves are vital foods. They contain the

power of germination still inside them and give the body maximum energy for minimum digestive effort. Fruits, when fresh or frozen, are likewise "alive." Unroasted nuts are potent, and of course all fresh vegetables, especially the green-leafed ones. And plain yogurt, with its live bacterial culture, is the best dairy intake.

Put all these together, and we have one of the most delicious breakfasts possible—and certainly the most healthy. The first step is to buy some fresh whole grains at a health-food store. A mixture of various small grains—red wheat berries, pearled barley, rye berries, millet—is best, and readily available.

Rather than grinding or cooking the grains, simply soak them for two full days in cool water (purified or spring water without chlorine is best). Rinse them morning and night, changing the water. Store them in water in the refrigerator after the second day if you're making a considerable quantity. Such soaked seeds taste extremely good!

Every morning, take a couple of large spoonfuls of soaked seeds and put them into a large bowl. Then add fresh bananas, oranges, apples, peaches, kiwis, whatever is available, cut into small pieces. Then add nuts (cashews, sunflower seeds, hazelnuts), whatever you like. Also raisins, if you want. The juice from a fresh orange is tasty to add. And finally, a serving of good plain yogurt. Mix this together, and you have superb Swiss müsli!

This breakfast is my recommendation for an ideal food intake in the morning. It should work for all illnesses except where more complete fasting is recommended. Some herb tea goes fine with this also. And certainly, if you need, some bread and butter as seems wise. And a poached or boiled egg once or twice a week.

If you are in the hospital, eating well becomes a problem. Do your best at least to get some grains soaking beside your bed, and insist on some plain yogurt daily if possible. When in the hospital, eating as little as possible is usually recommended. If you want further medical support in this regard, consult the books listed in the Bibliography, which will explain to your doctor the health value of such diets and fasting.

Lunch Suggestions

As a general rule, the best foods for lunch are fresh vegetables, cooked slightly in boiling water or a steamer, and a piece of bread. If you are going to have a small piece of meat, this is the best time of day to eat it. But let yourself become a little hungry, and you will find that the vegetables are suddenly extremely satisfying.

In fact, the trick of improving your diet is to eat only when you are very hungry. In this state, simple healthy foods satisfy completely. Only when you are eating too often do you need heavy meals to satisfy you.

And be sure that you don't let an overly motherly helper try to force food on you when you are not hungry. Let yourself be empty as much as possible. When we are in this empty state, both physically and emotionally, the great positive leaps of health tend to happen. To be sick and to have a full stomach is never recommended.

Dinner

For dinner, I strongly recommend a simple bowl of whole-grain brown rice as regular fare, prepared as you choose. If you are hungry, this will taste like candy! Too much has already been written about the value of rice as a regular diet (brown rice, that is), so I won't burden you with further praises. Whether sick or well, it is one of the best foods!

And whenever you want, a good soup is always a good food, especially if you make it yourself.

For drinks, fresh juices are optimum, if you have access to a juicer. Also, very often drink spring or deep-well water with a simple slice of lemon or lime; such a basic drink will evoke special feelings of simplicity and purity inside you. If you are seriously ill for a period of time, I strongly recommend getting a juicer, and making your own vegetable juices from raw vegetables. Carrot juice, beet juice, celery juice, wheat-grass juice—these have been praised for their seemingly miraculous healing potential. But don't become too faddish about any of these diets. To place all your hope and faith on, say, carrot juice, and to drink giant quantities of it—this would not be a balanced outlook on health. Instead, let good diet be a part of your internal healing process, balanced with the recovery sessions in this book, or other approaches you already find worthwhile.

Drugs While Sick

Basically, don't.

Caffeine, for instance, is nothing but bad news for a sick person. You don't want any artificial stimulants in your system, because after their brief stimulating effect, they inevitably drop you down even lower than when you started. Coffee and tea and cola drinks are addictions for many people. They run bodies down, so that infection and illness gain a foothold. Perhaps your sickness is simply a final reaction of your body to a too-large regular intake of coffee. See if you can do without it from now on. At least, notice carefully how it affects your vitality. Decaf coffee is an improvement, although the remaining acidic content is also a problem.

Also, beware of artificial sweeteners—I strongly recommend *never* using any of them. Real sugar is far better for your health, even though it has its own problems.

Nicotine is equally detrimental to the recovery process. Constant intake of this substance when you smoke can be a factor in the development of your illness in the first place. See if you can use this illness as a chance to stop smoking.

But please don't think that I am insisting that you give up coffee or cigarettes! I am only suggesting that you take a careful look at how these habits influence your health, and then act as you see fit. After all, perhaps you want to be sick, and the coffee and cigarettes are helpers in your campaign to ruin your health. I want to make suggestions about health in this book, not judgments about how you should run your life.

Candy and refined sugar and flour products, as you probably know, are also detrimental to the healing process. Illness is often caused at least partly by overconsumption of such "junk food." Usually, when a person falls ill, the stomach will not tolerate such bad food, and so the diet improves during the illness. How you alter your habits once you are well again is the critical question. Illness is similar to shifting a car's gear into neutral. In this open state, you can choose to shift your habits into a new gear that serves you better. Being knocked down for a while with a sickness presents a beautiful opportunity for change. What steps do you want to make next?

Alcohol? Overconsumption is, of course, not healthy for anyone. A general rule is, absolutely no alcohol while sick. But you must judge. Perhaps a glass of wine every couple of evenings is fine for you. But once again, chronic intake of alcohol is often related to final breakdown into illness. While you are ill, you can evaluate the way you use this drug as a habit, the effects it has on your life—and change gears if necessary.

In my opinion, marijuana as an occasional experience (once a month or less) seems to be relatively harmless to the health of the body. However, as a habit, it has been documented as reducing the body's resistance to disease. While ill, you should avoid regular use of hashish or marijuana. Perhaps the sudden insights that they may produce have helped people break free of old habits and move forward into health. But regular use of marijuana while sick generally makes people sicker. Specifically, it drains the body of vitamins, especially vitamin C, which is important for healing.

Cocaine has never been good for anybody's health and it will rapidly damage good health when used regularly. Indulging in it when sick is even more harmful. The same is true of amphetamines and barbiturates. Drugs in general do not improve anyone's health, and usually undermine it.

At the risk of upsetting your doctor, I will make the same qualified comment about prescription drugs. We tend to feel that our doctors should give us medication whenever we are sick. This has led to the terrible situation wherein doctors prescribe drugs more often than necessary, simply so the patients feel that they have "received some help."

But as most doctors readily agree, drugs are not usually the determining factor in anyone's recovery process. Recovery is an internal affair of your immune system. Most drugs have side effects that interfere with the bodily functions and tend to throw the body off balance.

I recommend that you let your doctor know you want to take prescription drugs only when absolutely necessary, and then in as small doses as possible. Ask to know the listed side effects of the drugs you do take. And, most important, don't rely on drugs to cure you, even if you need their help in extreme cases.

With all but the most severe fever, it is much better to allow a fever to take its natural course, than to take drugs to inhibit it. Fever is part and parcel of the healing process of the body. The experience of fever is a purification process; try to go through it as naturally as possible. Both a physical and a spiritual rebalancing usually take place with a fever.

Many miracle vitamin cures are being proclaimed today as the ultimate means of healing yourself. I have known people to recover from serious illness shortly after taking large doses of particular vitamins, but I could also see that their total belief in the vitamin cure might have been the active factor that generated the healing. We must be careful about cause-and-effect assumptions based on the sole evidence of obvious external factors.

So for vitamins: I recommend eating healthy foods that contain the vitamins we need. Sometimes an added supplement of particular vitamins and minerals can be helpful. But moderation is recommended. A healthy body eating healthy food needs no vitamin supplement.

Finally, I have a general recommendation about eating habits, one that is usually forgotten in such discussions. This has to do with when to eat, or more specifically, when *not* to eat.

Medical findings have shown that eating after six or seven in the evening produces a different digestive process from that produced when you eat during the day. Much of the food you digest while sleeping is not fully digested in the small intestine, but goes down into the large intestine and colon only partly digested. Here, an unwanted fermentation and bacterial decomposition takes place that actually sends toxins into your bloodstream. If you are a late eater and find that you habitually wake up feeling slightly nauseous, perhaps with a headache, this, more than alcohol intake, is probably the main cause of your morning distress.

These toxins are a further problem when you are sick. Your overworked system cannot deal with them. So I recommend strongly against eating after six o'clock. Don't let this suggestion slip by you unnoticed, because changing the time of your meals is something you can immediately alter to your advantage. Eat early, go to sleep early, wake up early—this seems best.

Television Stimulation: Healthy or Unhealthy?

The first introduction of television sets into hospital rooms was seen as a wonderful step forward: people lying sick in bed would no longer be bored and restless, but would be entertained.

Certainly the presence of "television energy" in a sickroom is acceptable as a minor, intermittent entertainment. But we should look closely at how television watching affects us before arriving at a more educated guess about whether television is healthy or unhealthy.

One observed effect of television watching is that it tends to reduce a full breathing cycle—in other words, people hold their breath a lot while watching television. This is partly because of the drama, which stimulates such emotions as fear, excitement, anger—feelings that are fine if they emerge naturally, but which, when overstimulated through television drama, inhibit relaxation and the calm state that is best for healing. When you watch television and generate a stimulation of your sympathetic nervous system, you are interfering with both the regular digestive functions run by the parasympathetic nervous system and your immune system's functioning. From this point of view, watching television while sick, at home or in the hospital, is definitely a negative influence on your recovery.

Watching television, of course, takes attention away from your state of ill health, and most of us want this avoidance when we're sick. From one point of view, this is wonderful. You experience your suffering less. Your conscious attention is almost totally gone from your physical body.

But think of our discussion thus far: you can see that watching television is directly counterproductive to your taking conscious responsibility for your own healing. If you came down with a cold and were home from work or school primarily because you were in need of a vacation, then sitting around watching television for hours while sick might be just what you needed. But if you genuinely want to explore the deeper purpose of your illness, television is perhaps the most counterproductive element in your environment.

I recommend strongly to all my clients who seriously want to improve their health that they allow no television at all in their room. Even the blank screen staring at you generates a conditioned response if you have been a television watcher in the past. At any moment, if you turn it on, the television may bombard you with radiation and light, stimulation and external distraction. As with any fond addiction, be it candy or cigarettes or television, if it is available, you will probably succumb to it—right when you are at an emotional crisis, which is also right when you are in a state to grow. If you turn on the TV at such a point, you lose a great opportunity for facing yourself and resolving inner conflicts and fears that, through your illness, are begging for attention.

Maximum functioning of the immune system occurs during a state of complete relaxation and minimum stimulation from the outside world. Watching the evening news puts you in just the opposite state.

So my general recommendation regarding television is this: when you are seriously involved with the healing programs in this book, and working consciously to explore yourself and your healing potential, avoid television stimulation completely. Either this, or in a more moderate attitude, watch only those programs that make you laugh and relax, brighten your day, and leave you feeling better than before you watched them.

But observe your breathing as you watch television. And if you find your breathing tense as a result of a program, it is best to turn off the set.

Music and recovery

As is television, music is an external stimulation of the senses and emotions. If healing requires relaxation, listen to relaxing music, keeping forays into rock and roll or heavy orchestration brief. Quiet meditation music is fine. You will find a special music tape listed in Supporting Programs (p. 181), which was developed directly to create a maximum state of relaxation and present-moment alertness, for encouraging the healing process.

I suggest that you don't listen overmuch to old favorite records and tapes, because this can serve as an opiate, rather than as a stimulus for growth. In general, silence is golden during illness. Stimulation that activates the sympathetic nervous system (loud and fast music) is detrimental; meditation music and the quiet classic pieces, optimal.

Reading while ill

Read what helps you relax, and avoid what makes you tense. And don't read for more than fifteen or twenty minutes without pausing to relax and tune into your body. As a general rule, short stories are better than long novels, because you return to the present moment more often. And be sure not to read novels that make you tense, or that stimulate unbalanced emotions. Choose only material that lets your breathing be free, your emotions expansive. Magazines such as *The New Yorker* often prove optimal, with diverse nonsensational reading adventures.

8

INTEGRATING PAST AND PRESENT

Our ongoing relationship with our past is a vital factor in our present relationship with ourselves and the world. Our present health and vitality, our living habits and dominant attitudes are all an expression of how past experiences influenced our development. Both the ability to be spontaneous and full of zest and the tendency to be contracted and in poor health are a result of our past. So our relationship with this vast universe we call memory can be critical in determining our health and our ability to recover lost vitality.

On a lighter note, looking back into one's past while sick can be the best entertainment in the world. In this Memory Balancing recovery session, we are not only going to delve into the deep dark blank periods of our lives where monsters lurk, but also into the beautiful times we have perhaps lost touch with, when we were full of energy and in robust health.

This means that we are going to seek a balance in our relationship with our past, a balance between wonderful, positive times and the more difficult, contracted times. As was our Emotional Balancing, this Memory Balancing is a key to a new sense of vitality.

Very often, we carry within us quite unrealistic concepts of what our past has been like. Some of us remember only the good times, creating a distorted notion that our past has been nothing but wonderful, whereas our present life is always less in comparison. Others of us do quite the opposite, remembering only the negative times we have had in our past and doing our best to escape from our past completely.

Such habits of memory create an imbalance in our self-image, which creates a further imbalance in our emotional energy, which finally manifests itself as a health imbalance and disease. Such patterns researched with cancer patients have showed a repeated lack of integration between past and present and a highly distorted concept of what actually happened in the past.

The challenge in this session is to put to use particular techniques to help regain a balanced and realistic concept of the experiences in our past that have influenced our development. At the same time, we are going to allow old experiential wounds to heal emotionally, so that they no longer generate denial and anxiety at unconscious levels.

To do this, we are going to take a leap of trust in the direction of the unconscious mind. My experience as a therapist has shown that human beings have a natural "homeostatic" process of memory balancing, just as they have a physiological homeostatic function that works toward balance in health. We are going to tap this "wisdom of the unconscious" through a very simple but effective technique.

As children, we often had experiences that frightened us or violated our developing concepts of reality. When this happened, we tended to blot from our conscious minds the memory of the conflicting experience. Thus we created blank spaces in our memories.

Unfortunately, when we want to repress a single hour of our past from our memory banks, we often blank out entire days, weeks, even months and years, in order to keep the unacceptable hour out of our conscious minds.

As we learn this technique for going back into our past on "rediscovery expeditions," we will find that we suddenly open up a vast reservoir of lost memories, just through opening ourselves to a single blocked memory of a single isolated experience. In this way, we regain a lost part of ourselves, and this recovery process can bring sudden and dramatic increases to our present vitality.

In the same way, we can go back and enjoy periods of our past that were pleasurable and positive and suddenly find ourselves remembering, with no difficulty, an experience during this time that was traumatic. When we see this particular experience in the balance of surrounding positive memories, we can easily accept and appreciate the trauma we experienced, and thus release ourselves from the denial.

The word *denial* plays a large role in the psychosomatic theater. When we reject parts of our past, we are in effect damaging our integrity at a very deep level. Most people who walk into my office are caught in this denial pattern. As long as this basic habit is active, there is very little hope of freeing needed energy for healing. In fact, illness is often a direct expression of the denial pattern.

In the Direct Focusing recovery session, for instance, you may have discovered that you rejected that part of your body that was sick. A denial pattern in a physical disease is usually the development of a more internal denial pattern of one's past.

People who claim, even to themselves, that they had a perfectly marvelous childhood, with no traumas whatsoever, are very often people who develop psychosomatic disorders—or even disorders not usually considered psychosomatic. Denial of either negative or positive results in a serious imbalance. Depressive people actively deny that there is anything positive happening inside or around them at all. But the imbalance exists equally in those constantly smiling "power of positive thinking" persons who refuse to open their experience to the more negative dimensions of life.

The opposite of *denial* is *acceptance*. This word, like *healing*, has been so overused that sometimes it seems to have no meaning to us at all. But I should like to put aside the various ways in which the word has been manipulated for special causes and take a look at the emotional, cognitive, and physiological, processes that the word represents.

When we accept something, we open ourselves to being influenced by it. We allow this something to exist with us in our world, we grant it space to live. We need make no effort to deal with things around us that we accept, because we are in harmony with them and can accept their influence on us. Acceptance means participation *with* something or someone; it means interaction.

Rejection and denial are shutting-out processes. When we reject something, we must act to eliminate this something from our world. We feel threatened by the influence of this something, and with this feeling of fear comes a reaction of aggression or of running away to escape from the influence of the threatening person or situation.

This aggression or running away requires constant energy, and this energy is energy lost to our biological and emotional systems.

What applies to present-moment acceptance or rejection applies equally well to experiences that have moved into memory but that still exist inside us and can have strong effects on our feelings and thoughts.

Thus, if a terrible experience threatened us deeply, violated our self-image and concept of the world, we may have reacted to it by rejecting the experience completely. We may still want to run away from the experience and the fear it creates when we think of it, and to run away, we try to blot the memory from our conscious recall.

This blocking of a past experience takes energy. People who deny great parts of their past are people who employ large amounts of their vitality to this process of blocking. They make themselves vulnerable to illness because of a loss of overall vitality and because their very act of running away tends to maintain the old sense of fear inside them. They know that if they ever let down their blocks, the feared experience will suddenly jump at them from memory; and the shock of this remembering, of reliving the dread experience, is something they fear and avoid at any cost.

In your present situation, perhaps such denial of part of your past is costing you your good health. I offer this only as a possibility for you to consider, as you explore this chapter's Guided Memory-Balancing Excursions recovery session. If you do have repressed memories that are still under pressure to come out, be remembered, then let go of and accepted, then you can use this present illness as your chance to do just that.

Regaining Your Childhood Spirit

Another beautiful dimension of this memory session is the opportunity to regain contact with the vital spirit you were born into this world with. Small children have a natural sense of personal power and vitality that is all too often repressed as they get older. A therapy technique that has proved effective for increasing immune-system functioning and resultant recovery of health has been one that helps clients remember the feelings they had when they were very young, especially the bodily feelings and breathing patterns that reflected their enthusiasm and openness to new experience.

Pause a moment right now and reflect upon your childhood. Can you make direct contact with how you felt when you were young? Is this early spirit still bright and active inside you, or has it somehow been lost through the years?

More directly: did you have some experiences when you were young that were so traumatic and negative that you have blocked your memory and contact with your entire early childhood, just to avoid the few experiences that threaten you?

The remembering of a past experience produces a quite marvelous, and at times frightening, experience in our bodies in the present moment. We find that we can relive a past experience, feeling in our muscles and our glands, our emotions and our perceptions, exactly what we felt when the experience actually happened to us. And it is this direct linkage of past and present, through the body, that makes the past so powerful to us in the present moment.

Some people are stuck in the past, in times when they were depressed and frightened. They carry with them into the present moment a constant state of contraction; they have developed a habit of fixating their attention on a particular memory or series of memories. By remembering a frightening past experience, fearing that something similar will happen in the future, they re-create a chronic state of anxiety. This condition is rampant in our society, and has reached such a level that to be anxious is almost the normal emotional state. People addicted to the news media, for instance, are usually caught in this past-present imbalance: always afraid that something terrible may have just happened and wanting to know about it.

I could carry on with this preliminary discussion for hundreds of pages, but it is more important to move on to the actual process of past-present integration. Your personal experience with the recovery session will show you what significance and power it has for you and your health.

RECOVERY SESSION EIGHT

Guided Memory-Balancing Excursions

You will want to set aside twenty to thirty minutes for this recovery session, if you want to go through the whole process at one time. The approach we are going to use employs a very gentle quality of hypnotic suggestion to help you move effortlessly into your past, without influencing the content or emotional qualities of your unique memory adventure.

As with earlier recovery sessions in this program, you can either read through the description of the session here, memorize it, and guide yourself through the process; or you can ask a friend to guide you by reading the description; or you can work with the professional guided session available (see p. 180 for description).

If a friend is reading this recovery session to you, the timing between each different category, when there is silent time for your remembering, should be between one and two minutes, as it is on the professional tape version. It is important that the words written here be adhered to faithfully, because they are specially chosen to elicit a deep, broad range of experience.

As we did with the Emotional Balancing recovery session, we are going to use elicitor words and sentences to point your attention in the right direction. There are twelve different memory categories that we are going to consider in this recovery session, each of which will awaken experiences you had in your past. This session can be repeated literally thousands of times without growing stale because you have such a vast memory bank of experiences inside you.

A crucial aspect of this recovery session is integrating the memories you have into your present-moment consciousness. After each memory category's trip into your past, you will want to return to the present moment for a few breaths, feel yourself here right now, and allow the experience of your past to integrate itself into your experience in the present moment.

This sounds simple, but it is quite a bold move to make regularly. Step by step, you will become quite adept at shifting from past to present. And then at a certain point you will find yourself making a radical discovery that runs quite contrary to our programmed concepts of reality but that is actually more realistic than the existing notions of time and space.

This discovery will be that there is, in fact, no real boundary or border between past and present. As you move freely back and forth between memory and present experience, you will find yourself in an expanded state of consciousness in which the feelings in your body are seen as coming simultaneously from both present perceptions and sensations and past perceptions and sensations.

We are always living in this integrated past-present reality: the separation is only an illusion of the thinking mind, which tries to separate memory experience from present-moment experience. Everything we do in the present moment, after all, stimulates our associative mind to remember similar experiences, and we find ourselves reliving past experiences while we are living this new experience for the first time. And then a moment later, our present experience has become memory itself!

Somehow, in ways that are not yet understood scientifically, this conscious integration of past and present serves to generate an increase in vitality in the body.

So, on to a memory adventure, to see what we find today!

First, sit or lie comfortably, notice your breathing, and let your eyes close when they want to.

Notice the air flowing in and out of your nose. Listen to the sounds around you. Feel the movement of your chest and abdomen as you breathe effortlessly. Let your breathing stop when it wants to. Notice your whole body at once, as you breathe.

Now remember, without any effort, waking up this morning in your bed. Let the memory come to you as it wants to. Remember opening your eyes. What did you see? What did you hear? What were your first thoughts and feelings this morning?

Now let go of that memory and be aware of your breathing in the present moment right now. Listen to the sounds around you, and relax your body. Feel the contact between yourself right here right now, and yourself this morning waking up. Enjoy this feeling of connectedness with your past experiences.

Now let yourself go back in memory to an earlier morning, when you woke up in a different bed. Let memories come effortlessly of waking up and experiencing the world around you, at some earlier time in your life.

What do you see when your eyes open in the morning? What sounds do you hear in the house? Let your memories expand and take you where they want to go.

Now let go of that memory, and return effortlessly to the present moment. Feel your breathing right now.

Allow your eyes to open for a moment and see the space around you, as you breathe effortlessly the air in the room.

Now close your eyes again.

Allow your mind to return to an earlier time in your life, to a day when you were swimming somewhere, or playing in water.

Remember the feeling of the water on your skin, as you splash in the water. Feel your breathing, and let your memory take you deeper into the experience of going completely into water over your head for a moment.

Now remember coming out of the water with the feel of the air on your skin.

Look around you and see where you are, if you are alone or with someone. And let the memory go where it wants to with you.

And now you can let go of that memory, and return for a moment to the present, as you breathe and feel your body right now.

Now go back in time again, remember being with a person you loved very much. Open yourself to whatever memory comes to mind effortlessly of an intimate experience with someone for whom you felt deep oneness and love.

Let the memory take you deeper into the reliving of this experience, and be open to whatever comes.

And now let go of that experience, and bring yourself into the present moment again. Breathe, feel your body in the here-and-now, and allow your eyes to open again for a moment. Look around you, feel yourself completely here. And now let your eyes close; relax; breathe.

And now allow yourself to go back in time, to a day when you were working. Let a memory come of being completely involved in work you were doing. Remember the experience of doing your job, performing your goal successfully. And see what memories come to you as you remember working.

Now relax and effortlessly return to the present moment, as you let go of your memory and feel yourself here in the here-and-now. Breathe, relax, notice the feelings in your body.

And now go back to a day in school. See where your memory takes you, open yourself to remember any experience related to schooldays.

Notice what schoolroom you are in. Who is the teacher? What schoolmates are around you? Remember the smell of the room. And let the memory take you where it wants to.

Now let go of that memory, notice your breathing here in the present moment.

And now let your mind return to a time in your past, when you were doing something with an animal, either one that you loved, or perhaps one that you were afraid of or didn't like. See what memories come as you remember this experience. Notice how your body feels in this experience, and let the memory take you where it wants to.

Now let go of that memory, return to the present moment. Watch your breathing. Let your eyes open for a moment. If you want, stretch your body and yawn, and then close your eyes again.

Now let yourself go back in time, to when you were playing with one of your very best friends in childhood. Let the memory come effortlessly. Enjoy the intimate experience of playing together, and see where your memory takes you.

Now let go of that memory, and come back to the present moment. Relax, hear the sounds around you. Watch your breathing.

And now let yourself return to a time when you were playing a game or sport in your childhood. Remember the feeling in your body as you played the game. Look around you and see where you are, and who you are playing with. And let the memory take you where it wants to.

Now just relax, feel your body here in the present moment, breathing, relaxing more.

And now go back in time, to when you were young, and doing something with your father or father figure. Open yourself to whatever memory comes to you, as you and your father share an experience together.

And now relax, let go of that memory, and return to the present for a moment. Open your eyes. Notice the feelings in your breathing, your body. And now let your eyes close when they want to.

And let yourself go back even earlier in your childhood, to a time when you were with your mother. See what memories come to you as you open yourself to them.
You and your mother, together.

And now just relax, let go of that memory, and return to the present for a moment. Notice your breathing. Your whole body.

And now let yourself go back in time to whatever memories want to come to you now. Be open to any experience you ever had in life, and relive whatever comes to you.

And now you can relax, let go of that memory, and slowly return to the present moment. Feel your body here, and your breathing coming and going effortlessly.

And when you are ready, you can open your eyes, and reflect upon what you just experienced in this session, and go on about your day when you are ready.

So now you see the general flow of the Memory Balancing recovery session. If you want, for yourself, you can also add other general types of experiences. But you will find that these twelve basic categories will open up vast realms for you if you go into them deeply.

As you can see, it is difficult to be bored while sick if you regularly let yourself go on such an adventure into your past. Through this structured experience you will find that your memory in general will begin to loosen up, to become more active and more willing to explore previously blocked memories.

You will, in essence, begin to regain yourself. You will rediscover the experiences that have made you who you are. And by reliving and accepting these experiences and reducing their emotional charge through this acceptance, you will become free of them, and able to move on more freely in the creation of your new moments and living habits.

The Memory-Balancing Recovery Session at a Glance

If you are doing this recovery session by yourself, you can open your eyes to glance at each new category and then close your eyes and go back into the experience.

Remember the following:

1. *waking up this morning in your bed*
2. *waking up in an earlier bed*
3. *a day when you were swimming*
4. *being with someone you loved very much*
5. *a time when you were working*
6. *a day in school*
7. *an experience with an animal*
8. *being with a best friend in childhood*
9. *playing a game or sport*
10. *experiences with your father*
11. *with your mother*
12. *any memories that come to you*

Be sure to pause in between each category, so that you integrate your memory experiences into your present moment. And make sure your breathing remains primary.

9

ATTITUDES
AND
IMMUNOLOGY

We now come to a discussion that strikes directly to the core of immune-system functioning and to our general level of vitality or ill health.

Have you ever noticed that some people fully expect to get a cold every three or four months? They will tell you that this is just their disposition: they are people who get frequent colds. They anticipate their next cold, and when it comes accept it as if it is their fate. They have, in short, a self-image of being a cold-plagued person.

Other people are accident-prone. They have had numerous accidents in the past, and they see themselves as somehow more vulnerable to accidents than the average person. They are apprehensive in their bodies, anxious that a new accident will happen. This very attitude generates the bodily uncertainty that leads to accidents.

As I was growing up on a cattle ranch in the West, stumbling around in oversize cowboy boots in my father's footsteps, I saw very early how a person's attitude would determine his ability to succeed in work and his ability to relate successfully with people around him. Some cowboys on the ranch had a positive, strong attitude about their ability to ride a wild horse, for instance. When they were bucked off, they would reject the defeat and climb back on until they had ridden the horse successfully. They constantly reinforced their self-image of being able to succeed.

On the other hand, there were the cowboys who were uncertain of their self-image. They were unsure of themselves in difficult situations and, based on bad experiences in the past, would approach a mean horse with apprehension. The uncertain cowboys were caught up in tensions and fears that directly undermined their success with hard jobs and thus got them injured most often. The more this happened, the worse their self-image became. It was a vicious circle: they would develop a constantly worsening self-image, and thus do worse and worse in their work, until Dad had to fire them, or they became disillusioned and went to town to find less demanding employment.

The situation with the Indians was even more dramatic. They could do the same work with cattle as did the white cowboys, but their attitude was light-years away. They did not see themselves as fighting against nature, as the white cowboys did. They were more integrated with nature, and went about their work in a softer, less violent way. But many of them had an attitude, a self-image, of being a defeated race, which undermined their ability to succeed in the new period of history in Arizona.

Thirty-five years later, at a recent medical conference in Switzerland, I met a doctor who had just returned from doing research on the very tribe that I had grown up among. I learned from this man that these Indians had the highest incidence of diabetes of any population in the world—nearly 40 percent. Medical research on these tribes had concluded that there were two primary factors leading to their seeming plague of diabetes. The first was their immense intake of carbohydrates and sugar; the second was their psychosomatic condition—namely, their sense of hopelessness and despair.

At the same conference, much mention was given to new research demonstrating a link between poor recovery rates with certain types of cancer and attitude structures. One of the studies, a ten-year investigation by King's College Hospital Medical School in London, found that women with a positive attitude toward recovery had a 70-percent survival rate ten years after breast-cancer surgery, while women with a fatalistic or hopeless attitude toward their recovery potential had only a 25-percent survival rate.

This is a dramatic statistical piece of evidence linking self-image, attitudes, and the immune system's success in maintaining health in one's body.

A look at cellular behavior in dealing with infection reveals a remarkable story that parallels what we have just been considering. For a number of years, biologists have known of the existence of tiny molecules that inhabit the surface areas of all animal and many plant cells. These tiny beings are called by the rather clumsy name *glycosphingolipids*, and until the last few years were mostly ignored by research because they seemed to serve no known purpose.

But recently it was found that these tiny creatures are often directly implicated in the development of cancer growths. This has sparked a fervent wave of research to determine who they are and what they are doing in their life upon the surface of cells.

What has been found is really quite exciting: these molecules actually are communication links among cells as well as between cells and such foreign invaders as bacteria and virus. Glycosphingolipids mediate cell-to-cell recognition and determine responses between the membrane of the cell and the outside world. They are also crucial in decisions regarding growth of cells in the body.

As long as the "attitude" of the glycosphingolipids living on the surface of a cell's membrane is normal, they tend to refuse communication and interaction with virus and bacteria invasions that enter the bloodstream. But when the attitude of the glycosphingolipids shifts, then an open doorway is provided for infection through the initiation of glycosphingolipid contact.

However, I do not want to make the glycosphingolipids into our enemies in general. They serve a vast positive function throughout the body, everywhere coordinating communication between cells. And in many cases, such as in the lining of the stomach and intestines, it is essential that friendly bacteria be welcomed into contact with cells through glycosphingolipids.

For infections to take hold inside your system, it appears that your glycosphingolipids must develop a changed attitude, an altered self-image that makes them play a role opposite to what they usually play in your body. Instead of saying to dangerous invaders, "No thank you, go away from this cell," they, for some reason as yet unknown to science, begin saying, "Well, hello there, how would you like to come inside this cell?"

With such a change in glycosphingolipid attitudes, cancer and the other infections that make up the majority of our illnesses are given the chance to attack us.

We now come to the heart of the matter. What is the relationship between a person's emotional and mental attitudes, and the attitudes of the glycosphingolipids in the body? For instance, cells that become cancerous seem to have returned to their embryonic growth state for some reason, and it now appears that the glycosphingolipids are responsible for this regression into an earlier phase of life.

Does this reflect a general prevailing attitude of the person with this cancerous growth, of a desire to reject and deny the present adult world and retreat back into the security and peace of the womb?

Scientific technology for exploring the relationship between mental attitudes, emotional states, and biochemical functioning is, unfortunately, still in its infancy. We are dealing only with the gross, observable aspects of our organism's functioning, with little insight into the more subtle energy flows of the body that seem to underlie the biochemical observations we have made to date.

But we can turn directly to the research mentioned regarding a woman's attitude and self-image, and her body's immune-system functioning in surviving breast cancer, to see that there is a direct link between attitude and recovery rates. With this association established, we can look to your attitudes regarding your health, and see how you can act to alter attitudes and self-image fixations that may be undermining your ability to get well.

RECOVERY SESSION NINE

Expansion of Self-Image

We are now going to explore your beliefs and attitudes related to how healing takes place. To do this, I want to use a special technique. I will ask you key questions, and instead of your instantly coming up with an intellectual answer, I want you to take a deep breath and allow your intuitive realms to be active in generating a response to the question. Be sure not to judge yourself if you suddenly find yourself thinking thoughts that might bother you. We all have several different layers of beliefs and attitudes inside us, and it is important to become conscious of old programmings that function mostly unconsciously and may directly interfere with our health.

So play with these questions. Read one at a time, then close your eyes or look away from this page, and see what comes to mind. Stay aware of your breathing, and let thoughts come to you effortlessly. Perhaps memories will be stimulated as well, or even fantasies.

Question one: "Who heals whom?"

Our modern scientific minds have quite a rational answer to this question. We know that our own immune system orchestrates our internal healing, that we heal ourselves. But when we are in the care of a doctor or a medical team, we often simply trust the doctor to perform the magic that makes healing happen, and look to outside stimulation for healing.

This question of who heals whom is deeply rooted in our cultural and religious traditions. In most religious beliefs, it is God who heals us, not we ourselves. We pray to God for help, and when we recover, we place the thanks for our healing on the greater spiritual powers of the universe, not on our own healing ability.

Where do you feel healing energy comes from? Does it come from within, from up above, or from down below?

Of course, most religions feel healing energy comes from above, and most people look upward for healing energy. The American Indians, however, consider this attitude quite curious, because for them healing energy comes mostly from Mother Earth. Christians, however, expect energy from this direction to be coming from the Devil. *What is your attitude? Do you expect to find earthly healing energy coming from down below, or do you expect contamination from the Devil?*

I am asking these questions because we all have many layers to our attitude structures and belief systems. You have a little boy or little girl inside you who believes one thing, and a more sophisticated adult that believes perhaps quite a different thing related to healing. When we fall ill and turn to healing ourselves, we often become caught up in earlier beliefs from our childhoods, beliefs laden with superstitious fears and fairy tales that generate conflict inside us.

The first step in resolving these conflicts is to see them clearly, to bring to the surface the old, outdated beliefs that are undermining your present efforts to heal yourself.

So reflect upon this question of "Who heals whom?" as long as you want to, and return to it several times during the next few days, so that new insights rise to the surface.

Question two: "Can you heal yourself?"

Try answering this question aloud a few times, and see what words come to mind. Let the different voices inside you speak freely; the ones that don't believe you can heal yourself, as well as the ones that are perhaps overconfident. Let a dialogue develop between the different attitudes you might have. "Can you heal yourself?"

Question three: "What would happen if you did heal yourself?"

If you stopped depending on outside help for healing yourself, if you let go of feeling like a victim and took full responsibility for your recovery—and if you then did recover quickly—how would your life be different? What would your friends think of you? How would your basic attitudes toward life change?

To take full responsibility for our own health is often a scary step for us. As long as we see ourselves as helpless victims, as children needing someone to come to our rescue, our role is simple. But when we assume an adult attitude toward our own health and take responsibility for healing ourselves, our entire attitude structure is transformed. We find ourselves face to face with many old attitudes toward work, love, relationships, and the like that also need to undergo a transformation.

Many of us were brought up in religious traditions that considered it a sin to feel we had healed ourselves. We were supposed to feel that God had done all the healing, and to thank him for this intervention in our lives. If we were raised in this tradition, and now start saying "I healed myself," even to ourselves, our old religious programming will react with a sense of guilt.

If, on the other hand, we are afraid to feel this attitude of "I healed myself," we may block the entire program outlined in this book. *Take a look at your old attitudes and beliefs. See if in fact they are undermining your present efforts to heal yourself.* Please don't think that this is a theological argument I'm raising. Theologians will almost always admit to both internal self-healing and to God's intervention in "cures." What we are dealing with are childhood fears, inhibitions as one aspect of a greater picture, the aspect called "I healed myself."

Question four: "Are there any positive aspects to your illness?"

There are almost always positive benefits that come with an illness or injury. Perhaps you don't have to go to work for a while, and this pleases the little boy or girl in you who sometimes doesn't like going to work at all.

Perhaps you receive extra love and attention when you are ill, or did when you were young. Many people are victims to the unconscious attitude that falling ill will bring a desired increase in affection and sympathy. Although we may be quite sophisticated consciously, we are often very childish in our unconscious attitudes, and these attitudes undermine our health in favor of emotional gratification. We will repeat this old sickness/compassion pattern over and over again, even if it no longer works for us in adulthood.

So just see what your mind comes up with as you reflect on what you are gaining through your illness or injury. Be honest, and let various voices speak. Remain aware of your breathing and the emotions that may rise to the surface.

Question five: "Are you using your present illness somehow to hurt someone?"

This question can be very hard to answer directly. I sometimes had this habit as a youngster myself, and I know it can be difficult to be honest when honesty disturbs our positive self-image. But remember that we are looking to find old attitudes that first need airing before they can be let go of. And we must first look without judgment if we are to generate a change in attitude.

A note of warning: Please be careful that you don't allow a renewed feeling of guilt to grab you if you find that you still harbor negative feelings inside you. To feel guilty is an almost total waste of needed energy when you are sick, because guilt for something you did in the past is yet another attitude that knocks at your self-image, and your resultant ability to heal yourself. We shall say more about this later.

Question six: "Are you somehow punishing yourself with your sickness?"

Do you feel, deep down, that you did something bad in your past for which you deserve punishment?

This is a harsh question to ask yourself, but please take a deep look and see if you can face the question honestly. Give yourself plenty of time to reflect upon this question.

Guilt is a terrible destroyer of health. I consider programming children with heavy guilt patterns related to "sinful behavior" to be itself sinful. It is a terrible way to condition children into obeying the rules of society. I find nothing spiritual at all in this kind of psychological manipulation. Children can be taught how to behave successfully in a culture without being burdened with guilt complexes that can ruin their health, vitality, and pleasure in being alive. Guilt is more a political programming than a spiritual one.

If you were programmed with a guilt complex that is even now unconsciously pulling you down, I hope you will open yourself to recognize this programming for what it is. *Are you in fact a bad person, deserving punishment? Is there no forgiveness in the world? And can you bring yourself to forgive yourself?*

Very often, to heal oneself, one must first forgive oneself.

What did you do that was so horrible that you deserve to suffer, perhaps even to die? Look back and see what you have done that was so terrible. Almost always you will find that what you did was not really so horrible, in adult perspective, as you once perceived it to be.

Only by looking back and directly facing those old memories can you bring them into the perspective of your adult views, and free yourself from the deadly judgments you may be carrying inside you.

Let me repeat what I said before: you must *relive* the experiences that generated your self-guilt and denial patterns. It is not enough to remember vaguely the "sinful" acts you committed. You must relive them to experience them fully, to discharge the emotions that you still hold inside you, so as to receive a new attitude and feeling towards the event. If you find that you still cannot forgive yourself for how you acted and what you did, then I strongly recommend talking this over with someone.

Question seven: "Are you ready to heal yourself?"
It is easy to imagine healing oneself sometime in the future. But what about your attitude toward action right now?
Breathe into this question, and if the answer that comes to you is "Umm, well, actually, not right now, just give me a little time . . . ," then accept this attitude, see that it actively postpones your recovery, and take a look at why you don't want to act, right now, to implement your recovery.

○

I hope that you will return to these questions a number of times. Let them reverberate deep inside you for the next few days, until you feel you have fully explored them.

Sentence Completion

There is another technique we can use to give you a direct view into your usually unconscious beliefs and attitudes. This is "sentence completion." I give you half of a sentence, then you complete it any way that comes spontaneously to mind. Each time you read through the first part of the sentence, open yourself to a new ending.

.

Read each sentence beginning, then take a good inhale and see what words come out of you to end the sentence. Give yourself the freedom to try many different endings to see which really reflects your deeper feelings. Don't be surprised if there are two or three quite different endings for each sentence inside you.

1. *"When I think about healing myself, I feel . . ."*

2. *"If I suddenly healed myself, my friends and associates would probably . . ."*

3. *"People who heal themselves are . . ."*

4. *"When I think about whether I am responsible for my own illness or injury, I feel . . ."*

5. *"If I healed myself, my self-image would . . ."*

6. *"The real reason I am sick is . . ."*

7. *"If I was well right now, I would be . . ."*

8. *"The funny thing about my sickness is that . . ."*

9. *"If I could forgive myself I would . . ."*

10. *"When I ask myself if I am killing myself, the first thing that comes to mind is . . ."*

11. *"When I think about the outside world, my first reaction is . . ."*

12. *"If you asked me if I really love myself, I would say . . ."*

After going through these questions, close your eyes for a few breaths and open yourself to whatever thoughts or memories come effortlessly to mind.

Gestalt Conversations

Yet another approach to opening up your attitudes to healing comes from the psychotherapy tradition of Gestalt. This technique, the *Gestalt conversation,* is related intimately to the Direct Focusing healing technique you learned earlier, and should help make that technique more powerful as well.

To have a Gestalt conversation, let yourself talk with the part of your body that is ill or injured. First, tell this part of your body how you feel about it. Let yourself express any emotions that are inside you regarding your sick part. If your back is causing you pain, for instance, go ahead and tell your back how you feel about the way it is hurting you. Blow off all the pressures you have inside you about this damned back condition you suffer from.

Then, once you have expressed yourself fully to your back, turn the tables and let your back speak to you. Take your back's point of view, and see what it would tell you about how you have been treating it all your life. At first this may seem silly, but as soon as you let yourself take your back's role, you will be surprised what your back has to tell you!

Do the same with whatever part of your body is the source of your suffering, inconvenience, and pain. Let the conversations go back and forth as you answer each other's accusations and attitudes, so that you find out what is at the heart of your relationship with this part of your body.

What most people find out through this procedure is that they quite definitely do not like the part of their body that is diseased or injured. After all, this part of the body causes pain and discomfort, and no one likes pain and discomfort. So the natural reaction is one of anger and rejection of this region of the body.

Of course, when we reject the part of our body that is sick, we are taking loving, healing energy directly away from that part of the body that needs loving attention the most.

Here we find a primary cause of poor recovery rates in sickness and injury. Our negative attitude toward the diseased part of our body creates a general emotional and physiological condition that counteracts the immune system's job of generating healing in the diseased region of the body.

By doing Gestalt conversations with yourself, you will unearth your unconscious attitudes toward this region, and begin to focus conscious attention on altering this unhealthy attitude. By taking the point of view of the sick or injured part, you gain compassion for it. This compassion will be the impetus for a growth in attitude toward this region of your body.

But be sure also to accept the childish reaction inside you that is angry at the pain-causing part. This is also a valid response. You will want to allow all the different feelings you find to coexist inside you together, just as you learned to allow your different emotions to coexist inside you at the same time in the Emotional Balancing recovery session. Such tolerance, such a widening of one's self-concept to include divergent attitudes, is a basic step in creating harmony and balance in your system.

With this sense of tolerance and balance comes the deeper physiological change that will bring an increased recovery rate. Please remember that this growth takes patience and bravery; in order to face what you habitually reject, you also need love, enough to allow all sides of you room to live. The childish side that hates what hurts you must learn to communicate with the intellectual side that understands the cause of the pain.

Self-Image and Recovery

Who are you anyway, really? As mentioned before, we all create a concept of who we are, based on selected past experiences. If our self-image is a negative one, if we consider ourselves unworthy in some way, and are therefore pulling ourselves down unconsciously through our illness, how do we go about reversing this self-image, which is a true danger?

We all strive to maintain a self-image. We identify with our concept of who we are, and perceive anything that endangers this concept as a danger to our very being. Our inner integrity is based on our sense of self, and this sense of self is based on the particular assortment of memories that we hold as our foundation for understanding who we are.

For personality growth to occur, an act of bravery is required. You must be willing to let go of your superficial self-image, so that it can be compared with the broader range of experiences that have in fact formed your deeper personality. To do this, you need to go through the Memory Balancing sessions already outlined, or a similar experience of opening yourself to usually blocked memories. You need to open yourself to emotional growth by surrendering to feelings you usually repress. Then you can begin to gain a deeper feeling for who you really are.

For instance, are you someone who deserves to heal and get well now, or are you someone who deserves to remain sick? And even if your disease is the natural last step in your life, and is a positive journey into the great beyond, are you someone who reacts to such new experiences with contraction and rejection, or are you someone brave enough to open yourself to whatever comes next in life, be it death itself, and to accept your evolution through life with both strength and the ability to surrender when needed?

Are you, ultimately, someone who can let go of your old self-image and, through the insistent pressure of your present illness or injury, evolve into a new being?

Death Itself

Books on health are not supposed to talk about death, but you know from the beginning of this book that our main aim in this discussion is to seek a healthy balance rather than to imprison ourselves in one extreme or another, which creates imbalance throughout our systems. So in talking about life and health, we should also talk about the reality of dying. For some of you, illness is a temporary phase of your normal life, a chance to shift gears, make new realizations, and prepare yourself for a new period of life. But for others, illness is quite possibly your pathway into the beyond. What is your attitude toward death?

To fight against death, to live as long as seems worthwhile, is our nature. But to deny the very possibility of death, to reject the fact that we will someday, perhaps quite soon, move into that ultimate experience of what comes after life—this denial can be the most serious mistake of our lives.

To live life because we are afraid to die—this is certainly hell on earth. We all fear the unknown, we all hate to let go of everything we have; but when this fear of a future experience undermines our present enjoyment of the moment, then the fear of death is a major detriment to our enjoyment of life.

When we fall ill, we naturally feel our mortality. Thoughts of possible death produce anxiety. At the heart of this fear, we so often find a self-image that does not really accept our coming death. This self-image sees itself as going on forever—though experience shows that at the physical level at least, life is of limited duration. Like all other things on earth, we too will pass away and make room for new generations.

So when we fall ill, and think that perhaps this is our time to die, we have an important opportunity to adjust our self-image so that it harmonizes with the fact that we are mortal, that our physical life will not go on forever.

Making this adjustment during illness often gives people a renewed sense of vitality in the present moment. After all, if you live in the future all the time, always looking forward to times ahead, then you are missing experiences right now. Illness brings into focus sharply the fact that the future may never come.

I belabor this point because in my work with sick clients I have found that healing seems to come most easily when there is a letting go of the future and an accepting of one's mortality. The resulting shift places primary value on the present, and less value on the projected future.

In this relaxed, accepting, yet vital enjoyment of the present moment, both healing and dying become dynamic. It is as important to have the right attitude when you die as when you heal. And I hope that you will use the programs in this book equally when it comes your time to die, as when it is your time to heal.

If you look to your breathing right now, what do you find? Did my talking about death make your breathing constrict? Or in fact do you have a self-image that accepts your eventual death?

Meanwhile, you can tell from your very breathing that you are alive. Movement is life itself. Your constant movements generate your inhales and exhales, the constant movements keep your heart beating and circulating your blood. These make up your basic experience of being alive.

And while we are alive, let us take advantage of this sense of movement that keeps us vital.

In our next chapter we look to the relationship between movement and physical health, movement and emotional health, movement and mental clarity. We have spent enough time in the realm of concepts. What about some action?

10

PERSONAL POWER
AND VITALITY

As in all other aspects of our lives, balance in terms of movement and rest plays a determining role in our overall health profile. Very often, people become sick because they have been chronically pushing themselves too hard and too fast, always on the move, and never pausing to relax and let their systems recover from their stress habits. And in the opposite direction, many people are underactive, avoiding exercise where possible, often becoming overweight as a result, and losing the basic vitality that underlies health.

So in approaching the question of optimal movement, both when healthy and when ill, we need to hold in mind this need for balance, rather than overindulging in extremes.

As children, we were masters of this balance. We were great movers when we were active. Every day, by nature, children run and play and push their bodies to their physical limits in terms of exercise. But also, children know instinctively how and when to stop their spontaneous movements, and to lie down and relax.

Regaining this natural balance between movement and relaxation should be our goal as adults, so that we have several periods of each day when we are active, and several periods when we take a break.

In a few pages we will discuss recovery programs for movement, once your health has improved enough for such whole-body action. But we need first of all to consider the question of movement when you are quite ill. And to begin such a discussion, we need to raise the basic question of personal power.

All of us are born with personal power. We have a vital life-force within us that maintains our energy levels at optimum functioning and provides us with a lifetime of personal power for manifesting our dreams and needs. I have written elsewhere extensively about this quality of personal power, because it lies at the heart of our adventure through life. In this book I want to place personal power in the context of a program for recovery from illness.

Illness is usually felt as a reduction in personal power. If this loss of personal power drops below a critical point, death may ensue. If your personal power begins to increase, you are usually on the path to recovery.

So we need to ask well-directed questions about how one can increase the level of personal power in the body. First of all, what are the physiological parameters of personal power? What makes us feel weak or strong?

This is a complex glandular question, determined by the capacity of the organs that secrete hormones such as adrenaline into the bloodstream, hormones that in turn activate the increase in muscular performance we associate with physical strength. Because these organs are controlled by master organs in the brain itself, and because these master organs are at least in part influenced by our emotional state, we find the heart of personal power to lie with our basic self-image and resultant thought patterns and emotional responses.

So once again, we find ourselves back to the question of self-image: a small person with a powerful self-image, for instance, can easily defeat a large person with a weak self-image.

If you are lying in bed feeling weak and defeated, with a negative self-image in which you are a helpless victim of infectious circumstance, you are directly undermining your level of personal power. Your overall vitality will be inhibited, and your healing potential kept at a minimum, in spite of the efforts of your immune system to fight against your illness. When self-image keeps personal power and vitality at a low level, healing processes are blocked.

Although there are many subtle levels of personal power that manifest themselves at mental and emotional levels, we will do best in this context to begin with the actual outward manifestations of personal power, to see the relationship between muscular activity and your life-force.

For instance, the movement of your breathing right now is an expression of your personal power. The same is true of your heartbeat. Pause a moment, as you have done before, and close your eyes after reading this paragraph, and watch the movements of your body as you sit or lie perfectly still. Make no effort to breathe, and observe your personal power manifesting in this life-sustaining movement.

RECOVERY SESSION TEN

Movement and Breathing Programs

You do not have to get up and run around the block in order to do movements that bring you into contact with your personal power. Even if you are totally unable to do any real physical exercises, you can experience your personal power in the movements of your breathing and heart muscles.

This then is our beginning point in using movement to increase your sense of personal power and to turn your self-image in the direction of increased vitality and healing potential. Do this passive-movement exercise regularly: experience your body moving effortlessly as you breathe.

As soon as you begin this "movement watch," you will find that your breathing begins to change. And in this natural change, which comes through the combination of your unconscious breathing habits and your conscious attention focused to your breathing, is to be found one of the essential techniques for increasing personal power.

We can now advance to a new level of movement in your body, this time generated by conscious participation in your movement potential. A few of you might be unable to do this, but for most sick people, this next exercise is both possible and invaluable.

Pelvic Awakening

The pelvis normally moves slightly with each breath we take, so that the breathing is a whole-body experience, charging the system with energy with every breath. But when we fall ill or are hurt, we tend to tense the pelvic region and to block any opening and release. Consciously reversing this tense holding pattern can bring a general surge of vitality into the body.

First, as you breathe, expand your awareness to include your pelvic region. Notice, right now, whether it feels alive or dead, weak or strong. Notice especially if it feels connected with your spine and legs, or if there is a feeling of disconnection in the pelvic region.

Now, very, very subtly at first, see if you can encourage your pelvis to move slightly as you breathe. As you inhale, arch your back a little, and let your pelvis rotate back naturally. And as you exhale, let your pelvis move forward with a touch of assertion in the movement.

As you do this, open yourself to the pleasurable feelings of the movement. Your breathing will tend to deepen, your chest expand and feel more powerful, and your whole body waken.

Do this only a few times if you have been seriously immobilized by your illness. But within your limits at this time, begin to make regular contact with the muscles that move your pelvis. Through this conscious action you can stimulate an increase in your personal power quite readily, breaking free of the unconscious tensions that have blocked your personal power.

Once you have done this pelvic movement a few times, pause, relax completely, and experience how your body feelings have expanded through this exercise.

Noticing how your personal power has changed after doing a movement is the essential second half of any movement program. If your self-image is to expand, you must bring to your attention new experiences that show your personal power to have changed for the better. Only with this new attitude toward your personal power will you develop an expanding self-image that maintains your personal power levels when you are not consciously working with the movements.

You will notice that these movements of the pelvis are similar to sexual movements, as well as to movements of assertion and anger. Personal power is a general muscular pattern in the body, which then manifests itself according to your momentary emotional and interpersonal situation.

Sensuality Excursions

When sick, we tend to shut down the sensual sides to our personality. Pain does not go well with sensual pleasure. And illness is not usually associated with a feeling of enjoyment in the body.

But I would like to reverse this attitude toward sensuality and illness, because tapping positive feelings in your body, either through the movements I will show you now, or through memories and fantasies that wake up pleasurable sensations in your body, can bring a rapid increase in your vitality and healing progress.

Movement of the pelvis is one approach to stimulating a flow of positive energy through the body. But you can also do subtle movements of other parts of your body to bring a renewed rush of connection and pleasure to this region.

Naturally you will need to limit your movements to match your physical condition, but I think most of you will be able to do the following:

1. *Roll your head from side to side gently, and feel this movement in an enjoyable way. You will want to approach all these movements with the intention of increasing positive feeling in the particular region of the body involved. Head movement can loosen up a stiff neck, for instance, and also awaken your equilibrium center through movement.*

2. *Relax your jaw, open your mouth as you move your head, and, if you want to, make a soft* ahhhhhhh *sound of pleasure. Inhale deeply, and then let a great spontaneous yawn come out of you, if this feels good. Yawning is one of nature's ways of releasing tensions throughout the body and should be encouraged as often as possible for people who are ill.*

3. *Move just the fingers on one hand, while the rest of your body is relaxed. Then raise your hand a little and shake the hand at first gently and then more vigorously, to release tensions in the fingers and wrist. Do this with both hands, enjoy the sensation. And do this quite often every day so that tensions do not accumulate in your hands.*

4. *Now tense the toes of one foot, and move that foot around as much as possible, to free the ankle of tensions. Tense the whole foot tight, and then relax. Do the same thing with your other foot. And then shake one leg, relax. Shake the other leg, relax.*

5. *Now try shaking your head quickly as if saying no with the movement. And say out loud, if you want, while you do this, "No, no, no, no, no!" Enjoy this expression, which is an early personal power movement of young children, and which will wake up inside you a playful, assertive strength. All too often, especially*

*when we are flat on our backs with a sickness, we feel we
are victims, unable to say no to anything. This movement will release tensions created by our dependent
condition.*

These are just a few suggestions for movements that are
possible even if you are ill in bed. What you should do for
yourself now is to play with this idea of moving regularly
in such a way that makes you feel good somewhere in your
body. Even if you have considerable pain, see if you can
find a particular movement or series of movements that
give you a momentary rush of pleasure in your body.

Exhale Energy

An additional technique for increasing vitality in the
body involves another aspect of your breathing. As mentioned earlier, fear and weakness are manifested by shallow breathing high in the chest, with the breath held after
the inhale. What might happen if you did the opposite of
this?

As masters of martial arts and sports know well, a
slow, controlled exhale is in fact the breath of power. And
holding your breath while empty generates a surge of
increased energy potential in the body. You can put this
ancient wisdom to work immediately with the following
exercise:

*Exhale slowly through the mouth, making a slight,
barely audible* ahhh *sound in your throat, a whisper
sound. Open your mouth quite wide, as if to bite. This
will awaken a feeling of power in your jaw muscles.*

*Exhale until you are completely empty of air.
Tighten your stomach muscles to push all the air out,
and then hold these muscles tight a moment, while you
are empty. Experience this empty feeling—it will open*

gateways to increased vitality, often remarkable sudden rushes of power and new hope.

Then when you are actually hungry for air, relax the stomach muscles and allow the air to rush into you effortlessly.

Then, at the top of your inhale, to balance the breathing, also hold the breath a moment.

Now again, exhale slowly, through the mouth, hold completely empty until hungry for air, then inhale quickly through the nose, hold a moment. Repeat this breathing four to eight times.

Now completely relax, make no effort to breathe, and notice how your personal power has been affected by this exercise.

The first few times you do this you may feel dizzy, or a little anxious that you aren't getting enough air. But play with this exercise enough times so that your conditioned reactions are overcome, and you will gain a new feeling of personal power.

I recommend doing this exercise at least once an hour for the duration of your illness, unless your special health condition makes it impossible. Don't force the exercise by holding your breath too long. Do it so that it feels good, and it will do wonders for you.

Muscle Power

It is important, especially if you are sick in bed, to feel your muscular power regularly. Otherwise, your self-image erodes as well as your muscles themselves. I recommend a regular routine of tensing various muscles in the body to give a feeling of power and to maintain muscle tone.

The trick with such exercises is to combine breathing

with muscular contraction. *For instance, tense one fist, and exhale slowly with the "breath of power" I just taught you. Then as you inhale, relax the fist completely. On your next exhale, tense the fist tightly again, and feel your power both in the fist and in your belly, the power center.*

Go through this tense/relax/tense/relax routine for four breaths, then totally relax and notice how the energy level in your body has been altered.

As you experiment with this muscle power exercise, you will find just the right amount of tension to apply each time so that you do not overexert yourself and make yourself tired. Do this within your limits at the time. If you are very sick, you will have only a little amount of personal power to work with, so don't overdo the exercises.

Your aim is to feel the power you still have in your body. Work with any muscles in your body that you want to in this manner (tense-exhale, then relax-inhale). Find the proper balance for your condition, and regularly reinforce your sense of personal power!

Fantasy Power Excursions

There is a basic path for using the imagination to stimulate a feeling of power inside you. By remembering times when you felt powerful, in reality or fantasy, you will stimulate muscular and glandular behavior in your physical body at a subtle level and enhance your present self-image as well.

Go back in your memory to times when you were full of personal power. Set aside time regularly to remember these incidents when you acted in a powerful manner. Also remember adolescent fantasies of being someone famous, powerful, successful. Tap into those early fantasies of being an ideal superhero.

Up and Out

If you are able to walk, let this section of our discussion be a strong suggestion to do so. Of course, you will not want to expend more available energy than you have. It is important to become conscious of your energy reserves, and not to overextend them. But it is equally important to put your energy to use by moving.

Walking is one of the best therapies. Human beings are walkers. Birds fly and fish swim; we walk. Not to walk for a period of time puts us out of touch with our basic nature. To regularly walk outside is always healthy.

If you cannot physically get out and walk, you can still walk in fantasy and memory. Remember that when you imagine a physical activity, your muscles subtly respond, stimulating your whole body. So go on regular fantasy strolls, hikes, swims—whatever comes to mind.

Whole-Body Movement Program

If you are able to do a regular movement program, there are a number of possible routes. First, you might want to see what yoga classes are available in your area, because *hatha yoga* (physical postures and movements) is one of the most refined total programs for awakening your body, and has proven valuable in innumerable healing stories.

Each person has a particular attitude toward movement programs. Some of us hate being told to do exercises because we had such negative experiences earlier in our lives with controlled programs. For those of you with this attitude—please, create your own!

For those of you who would like guidance, I give here a brief description of one movement program.

SHAKING. *Stand comfortably and shake your hands for a moment. Raise your arms in the air until you are on your tiptoes. Then lower your arms and shake one leg, standing on the other foot. Reverse and shake the other leg.*

Now shake your whole body at once, feet on the ground. Make some crazy AAhhhh! *sounds as you shake your head, and enjoy!* (Be sure to do these exercises with full awareness of how your breathing changes as you do them. Feel your personal power changing, self-image expanding as well.)

JUMPING. *Move directly from shaking into jumping. Breathe through the mouth, keep making crazy sounds, and let your shoulders be relaxed. Jump in a circle in one direction, and then reverse.*

PERSONAL POWER PAUSE. *Now stand quietly a moment with your eyes closed; breathe through the mouth until your breathing calms down. Then expand your bodily awareness by going through the first recovery session we learned in this book, in Regaining the Present Moment:* breathing/heartbeat/balance/whole body. You will certainly find your heartbeat this time, after jumping! And balance feels very strong when you are standing. Thus, you find yourself totally in your body.

Now allow your eyes to open and, as you become aware of the space of the room around you, say air *to yourself. Finally, to make the awareness of reality total, say* earth *to yourself, and expand your awareness to include everything earthly around and under you. In this state, you are totally here, with your power, in the present moment.*

UPSIDE DOWN. *Now bend your knees a little, bend forward until your hands are flat on the floor in front of you. Have your feet fairly wide apart and facing straight ahead. Breathe deeply in this position, and notice how your personal power rises quickly in this stress posture. Be sure to do this exercise in a way that you enjoy, so that you have an inner smile throughout.*

Now shake your hands and arms as you remain bent over. Shake your head also, and make wild, crazy sounds, with your tongue sticking out to discharge tensions in the throat.

Now with eyes closed, slowly stand upright. Breathe, and feel how this exercise has affected your personal power.

RUNNING POWER. *Let yourself walk slowly at first around your room, breathing through the mouth, then start running with short, light steps, lifting your knees high so that you quickly charge your body with power.*

Be sure to stop when you want to; never push yourself. And when you stop, pause and breathe freely.

FREE DANCE. *If you want a final step to enhancing your vitality, put on your favorite dance music, and let your body move as it wants to for as long as you want to.*

With these movement exercises you can quickly charge your body and enhance your health profile. Only five minutes are needed to totally alter your vitality.

My advice is to set aside five minutes a few times a day to do movements, if your health allows. But if you don't want to move, spend the five minutes "watching yourself not doing the exercises." This way, you will gain insight into the parts of you that are blocking healthy movements.

If you want help, certainly get a cassette (see Supporting Programs, pp. 178–81) that guides you through a program. Often an encouraging voice is enough motivation to overcome our inertia.

In sum: Movement is life. Stiff joints and unused muscles are an expression of blocked or reduced personal power. So see what you can do to move more.

11

INTUITIVE ACTIVATION TECHNIQUES

I should like to share with you now, to round out our discussion on immune-system activation, some of the more spiritual approaches to healing as taken from four of the world's primary religious traditions. You can try each of them in turn, and see how they affect your consciousness and physical condition.

The first technique comes from the American Indian tradition, whose healing techniques I have been studying for some time. In this healing meditation, the basic thrust is to gain healing power from the earth from which we all come.

The second technique comes from the Taoist and Zen traditions of China and Japan, traditions that have been extremely important in the development of these programs. They are quite pragmatic, relying predominantly on direct experience rather than on conceptual notions of healing. At the heart of both is the understanding that life is a flow in which we all participate. If we are, by nature, participants in this ongoing flow of life on the planet, there is really no effort we can make to break free of our present situation, except by first surrendering to the reality in which we find ourselves. Once this surrender and acceptance happens, then we can align ourselves with the powers of nature, and thus encourage healing to take place.

This is the opposite of most modern Western notions of life. In the West we are taught that life is a constant struggle, that we must battle against negative forces in order to survive. With this attitude, we very often "muddy the waters" of healing by keeping ourselves hyperactive mentally and emotionally.

The Taoist and Zen approach to sickness begins instead with a relaxation of all efforts to "escape from our present condition." Instead there is a quieting of all struggling, and a total unjudging perception of the existing situation. Through this calm centering process the body is freed of anxious confusions of the mind and can carry on with healing as best it can.

The third healing meditation of this chapter comes from the Tibetan tradition of Tantric yoga. In this meditation, we are going to draw into our bodies the healing power of the universe through what is called *light meditation*, a process that uses visualization, along with direct bodily awareness, to generate a powerful experience of being filled with healing light. Many people choose this as a primary technique for healing, and you can see if it is well suited for your personality.

The fourth meditation, from the Christian tradition, is a technique you can do with a friend who is interested in helping you with your recovery. You will want your friend to read at least this section of the book before doing the meditation with you.

The meditation is similar to the Hand-Directed Integration recovery session you have already learned, in that the hands are going to be used to focus healing energy where it is needed in your body. The technique is called by the traditional Christian name of "laying on of hands," and has its roots in the early days of the Christian community. You may find this especially meaningful if you and your friend are from a Christian tradition.

You will see that these four techniques are really very similar to the ones you have learned already in this program. Healing is healing. Many paths lead to increased immune-system functioning and bodily repair, but the primary process is always the same. By expanding your consciousness to break free of constricting attitudes and emotional tensions, then focusing attention on the healing that needs to happen, you open yourself optimally to whatever healing powers exist for you in the present moment—be they purely biochemical, as some believe, or also supported by the mysterious spiritual forces of the universe. What is important is to prepare yourself for the ideal state of mind and body in which your natural healing process can best function.

RECOVERY SESSION ELEVEN

Spiritual Healing Meditations

For each of these techniques, you will want to prepare yourself first with the four-breath, Present Moment meditation. With each new exhale, say to yourself, *breathing*, then *heartbeat*, then *balance*, then *whole body*. Throughout the meditations, keep your breathing as your primary focus of attention. If you do not do this, you will almost always drift into thoughts and memories, and lose the power that comes when you are fully here.

1: Earth Healing

You can do this recovery session by itself, or paired with the Hand Integration and Direct Focusing sessions you already know.

For Earth Healing, lie comfortably on your stomach. Make sure you are in touch with your breathing in the present moment, then do the following: place one hand with your palm on your forehead, then place the other hand with your palm over the first hand. Now simply lower your head down to the floor.

Arch your neck enough so that your nose is not touching the floor, and find the ideal position for your arms so that there's no stress. Be sure your legs are comfortable: move them and loosen any tensions in the muscles.

In this position, say to yourself, "Breathing/heartbeat/balance/whole body"; experience yourself in contact with the earth under you. Then say the word healing *to yourself a few times, on each new exhale, and see what experiences come to you as you continue to watch your breathing and to feel the earth under you.*

Don't anticipate anything "happening." The nature of all healing work is to provide a new experience, one you have never had before. Anticipation (which is always based on past experience projected into the future) is completely counter to the state you want to be in. Your breathing and the posture will guide you effortlessly into whatever experience you are ready to have.

The earth is a powerful electromagnetic force field, and scientific understanding of this force field is extremely primitive. What you are doing with this meditation is opening yourself to receive whatever life-giving energy may emanate from the earth to you—if you are responsive. This position usually generates deep relaxation as well as energy sensations in the body. Without thoughts, you can experience what happens naturally. This in itself is adequate for encouraging healing. We do not know the deeper wisdom of the technique. But we know it can be very powerful.

After perhaps six to ten breaths in this position, open yourself to any thoughts or images that may start coming to you in this posture. If you stay centered in your breathing as the thoughts and images start to come, you can have a deeply rewarding experience that may shed light on which steps you are ready to make in your life.

Then, sit up when you want to; and when you are ready, slowly allow your eyes to open, and carry the experience you just had with you to support your general healing process. Even if you are quite sick in bed, this meditation is usually possible, and is highly recommended. Try it now if you want to:

○

2: Zen Surrender (Nowhere to go, nothing to do)

For this meditation, first lie or sit comfortably, and do the four-word Present Moment meditation.

Then, with your eyes closed, as you exhale, say to yourself, "Nowhere to go." Put all future thoughts aside. Let yourself feel that at this particular moment you have no obligations to go anywhere or to move at all. You have the freedom to relax completely and not feel the habitual pressures of life that always keep us tense, the feeling there is somewhere we need to be.

With your second exhale, say to yourself, "Nothing to do." At this particular moment, nothing is required of you, no action, no work. You are completely free to do nothing, to go nowhere, to be yourself, at peace in the present moment.

In this state, chronic anxieties can vanish, habitual tensions recede. A sudden flood of energy can flow through the body, a warm sensation of expansive space and love. Or, of course, sometimes nothing at all will seem to happen. The Zen meditation state is not a great spectacular event, but rather a total harmony with the natural flow of life.

This is a state not only of accepting your own condition, but of allowing your attitude to shift so that you feel that you are also accepted by the universe in general. You are okay just the way you are, without having to make any effort.

In our childhood we are, all too often, reinforced for "doing something" rather than "being ourselves." This conditions us always to be busy doing something—and when we come to a complete stop, we feel anxious, uneasy, uncertain about our status.

Zen meditation generates exactly the opposite feeling: that of relaxed surrender. Such a feeling of surrender is often associated with a turning point in a person's illness. Until such a surrender is experienced, anxieties and tensions constantly interfere with your recovery. But once you relax and accept your present condition totally, opening yourself to whatever is happening to you, then small miracles, and even big ones, sometimes happen.

This "surrender" meditation is extremely simple, so

simple that many people reject it as not being sophisticated enough to have any power. What do you think?

As a final step, you can also, if it comes naturally to you as you do this meditation, say the word healing *to yourself as a third verbal cue, and simply let the word reverberate through your system, without any expectations. Let your breathing guide you into this beautiful experience. Go ahead and do this healing meditation now if you feel ready:*

O

3: Light Meditation

You can either memorize the basic flow of this meditation, and do it entirely on your own, or use the help of a friend or a cassette's guiding voice to talk to you.

Lie comfortably, preferably on your back, and close your eyes. Let your breathing come and go as it wants, stopping when it wants to, completely free and effortless.

Feel your body on the bed or floor, and notice where your body is actually touching the ground, so that you feel complete contact with the earth under you.

Roll your head from side to side a few times to loosen your neck. Open your mouth and make a soft AAhhh sound as you turn your head. Let your breathing deepen.

.

Now exhale completely and hold your breath a moment, before letting your next inhale come effortlessly. Do this breathing pattern a few times: Exhale, hold, inhale, hold, exhale, hold, inhale.

Let your breathing be completely free to come and go as it wants. Feel free to open your mouth and yawn a couple of times, tensing and stretching your body freely as you yawn, so that all your tensions are released from the body.

Now massage your face a little, as you continue to make soft sounds and release any remaining tensions from your breathing and body.

Now just relax completely. Make no effort to breathe. Feel your breathing, your heart beating, your whole body at once, completely at peace.

Now begin to imagine that a soft, warm, wonderful light is beginning to flow into your body, up through the soles of your feet. Feel your feet filling more and more, so that they become immersed in warm pure light.

Allow this light to continue to flow into your body from its infinite source in the universe. Feel your legs filling with light, warm and vibrant, flowing up your body with loving, vital energy. With every breath allow more light to flow up through your body, until you feel that your legs are completely filled with light. Relax your jaw and tongue, and let your breathing bring in more and more light into your body with every breath.

Feel this wonderful, healing energy flowing brightly into your pelvic region now, filling your creative, sexual center with warm, vibrant light.

·

And feel this energy moving into your belly, into the power center of your body, filling this region with pure warm healing light.

Feel the light flowing from your feet, up through your legs, through your pelvis, into your belly and lower back, and now flowing up your spine and into your stomach, filling you with light until you are immersed in healing energy.

Now feel this light filling your chest so that you are breathing the light in and out of your lungs. Let your heart fill with light, so that the blood throughout your body is radiant with healing energy.

Now let the light flow up through your shoulders and neck, effortlessly with every breath, flowing up your spine and into your tongue, your lips, your eyes, and finally filling your brain itself with healing energy.

Relax completely as this energy and light flows effortlessly through your body, bringing healing energy to every cell. With each new breath, feel the flow of light carrying away your illness and bringing you renewed vitality and health.

Now, when you are ready, allow your eyes to open. Stay with your breathing.

And when you are ready to finish this recovery session, carry the healing light with you, healing yourself with every new breath.

4: Laying On of Hands

Your friend may want to do the earlier healing meditations in this book first—especially the Hand Integration recovery session—to get in tune with our general approach to healing.

For this recovery session, the first step is for both of you to do the four-word Present Moment meditation, bringing you into a congruent time/space harmony.

Then both of you can lie down on your backs and do the Hand Integration session, to tune your hands into your own bodies.

After this, have your friend sit beside you (while you stay on your back), and take a few deep breaths along with you, breathing at your rate, so that you tune deeper still into each other's body rhythms.

Now, without expectancy, your friend will put a hand over the part of your body that needs healing attention. Eyes closed is usually best, as you both focus on contact of hand and body. Both of you will want to say to yourselves the word healing *a few times. Then just breathe, and experience what happens.*

You do not want to take a recovery session such as this too "seriously." Instead, do it lightly, with a sense of play even, so that your attitude is free of expectancies and anxieties. This is a very deep tradition you are tapping into. You probably have heard tales about healing sessions like this, tales filled with who knows what sort of drama and superstition.

So I suggest that you experiment with the recovery session in a casual way, remaining open to what experiences come to you, but not pretending to be caught up in a primordial ritual. This is at heart a simple focusing exercise. You are both helping your body to focus healing attention where needed. This in itself is valuable.

Often, of course, people do feel a flow of healing energy going from the helper's hand into the body of the ill person. Sometimes the experience of the Light Meditation comes spontaneously into this "laying on of hands" session, and a beautiful flow of light is experienced.

Also at this point, if you are of the Christian religion, you can call on any form of prayer to tap into the healing power of the Holy Spirit.

I hope you can see my reason for putting all four of these spiritual healing meditations together in one chapter. Together they make a "whole." Each adds a particular dimension to the overall healing experience; they balance each other. So you might want to take these four meditations as a unit, and do them together. Of course, when a friend is not available, you can do the Hand Integration healing session as the fourth meditation, since it is, in essence, a solo version of the "laying on of hands."

Strong emotions very often come to the surface when you do such meditations. Please always open yourself to these emotional flows, rather than block them because they are disturbing your meditation. Emotional healing is just as important as physical healing, and usually the emotional discharge comes first. So do not block feelings. Instead, breathe through the mouth, let your emotions come out.

12

SURVIVING A HOSPITAL EXPERIENCE

None of us likes to spend time in a hospital, but there are times when it is unavoidable. When you do find yourself flat on your back in a hospital bed, at least there are ways to make the best of a trying situation.

I should admit that I have never been hospitalized, so I cannot speak firsthand of the experience. But I have known hundreds of people during their hospital stays, and have gained insights by helping them with their period in hospital. I hope the suggestions in this chapter are of value to you if you are in a strange bed in a strange room, with strange people doing strange things to you during this strange period of your life.

If falling ill generates anxiety, then having to go to a hospital generates still more. We all know that many people go into a hospital and die there. Let us look directly at this fact, because it causes great emotional turmoil when pushed down into the unconscious and not faced.

My advice is to talk openly about this anxiety with someone. I was for a time a minister working for a large church, before I returned to secular work, and one of my main jobs was doing hospital rounds. And I found that if I gave patients the chance to voice their anxieties about being in the hospital, they would break free of the tensions this anxiety was creating inside them.

All too often, patients try not to upset their friends and loved ones by expressing negative feelings while in hospital. But I recommend the opposite. Your friends are in a better position than you; let them carry some of your emotional burdens now and then. If they want you to recover, they should understand that you will recover faster and more deeply when given the chance to express your apprehensions.

Often I would bluntly ask a patient if he thought he was going to die. This might be considered unkind, but it worked in exactly an opposite way: the patient was relieved that someone had finally asked him the question that was creating unknown suffering inside him. Once all the talking and perhaps crying or anger was expressed, the patient felt greatly relieved.

So don't try to be the strong one when you're hospitalized. Instead let your weaknesses show, express your fears and apprehensions, get them off your chest. This is the best path to health. If certain friends don't want to help you, they needn't visit you. You need people around you who help, not hinder, your healing.

Healthy Connections

Illness is often an expression of broken contacts, of a lack of healthy connections with the outside world. When you are in the hospital, consciously open yourself to other people, if your energy is up to it. But don't play the usual social games. It is tiring and usually fruitless to hide behind a false mask.

Instead see if you can watch your breathing when someone is with you, and stay in touch with your deeper feelings. Let the present moment be your growing ground. Try to relate on a deeper level, if only with your eyes as a beginning. Be honest. This will create unexpected flows of vitality in your body. Risk letting people see how you feel, even if you feel bad. Often we keep ourselves ill because we block honest contact, thereby cutting ourselves off from the nurturing energy of human compassion and communion.

If you have long periods with no visitors, you can do some of the Memory Balancing sessions we have explored already, and remember people you have been close to in the past. Give yourself that feeling of human contact that helps to encourage healing.

Let insights come to mind as you reflect upon your old social habits. Look at your living habits to see where you may have been inhibiting the very type of interaction you need in your life.

I cannot go into a lengthy discussion of interpersonal needs here, but this factor can be very important in a person's health. When we are isolated and cut off from others, we tend to lose vitality. Human beings are social animals as well as solitary beings, and we thrive on healthy connections with others. If you feel this is a problem in your life, let me point you toward the book I've written on this subject, *Finding Each Other,* which offers a full program for reaching out to make contact with the types of people you need deep-down.

Hospital Attitudes

We tend to feel like victims when we are hospitalized. We are treated like helpless dependents in most large hospitals, with our normal sense of independence suddenly stripped away. We even lose our regular clothes and personal habits, and are subjected to many types of treatment that would evoke anger under normal conditions.

I have often wondered what would happen to a healthy person who was suddenly forced into a hospital bed and subjected to the hospital routines for a week or two. This experience is a shock in itself and you must consciously deal with it so that it itself does not further undermine your health.

You are, for instance, surrounded by sickness in a hospital. The very smells remind you of illness, and usually the food is extremely lacking in vitality. Often doctors look at you with that superior attitude that comes when one spends all day relating to people flat on their backs looking up at them helplessly. Your uniqueness and personal worth are lost amid the hospital routine, by the very nature of a hospital organization, by the processing of patients day after day, year after year. You have just replaced someone who was sick in your bed before, and there will be someone new to replace you when you are gone. To expect the staff at a hospital to be other than they are is unrealistic. They too are doing their best in a difficult situation.

So how do you deal with a hospital environment that constantly places you in a sick, weak, helpless role? First, as just mentioned, do all you can to establish healthy relationships while in the hospital, both with other patients, the staff, and friends who visit you.

Second, busy yourself with the various sessions I've outlined, so that you reinforce your sense of personal power and responsibility, and counteract the opposite pressures around you. Make sure you do what you can to exercise, even if it is only a slight tensing of your muscles. Eat as well as possible. And face your fears and worries consciously.

You also have a vast opportunity to explore your inner worlds while you are in a hospital. Do your best to receive as few mind-blurring drugs as possible: be firm with your doctor that you want a minimum of medications. Use your clarity of mind to grow, to help yourself heal, to entertain yourself through inner trips and exercises.

A "Walkman" tape player can be of great value. Classical and other relaxing music is very helpful. And if you want, use the cassette programs described on pages 178 to 181. Perhaps your hospital already has these in stock, or you can request rapid handling if you order them directly. Having a voice to guide you professionally and lovingly through the recovery sessions is of immense value when you are struggling to hold your own in a difficult environment.

Guided fantasy adventures can be rewarding as well as pure escape and fun. The one I am going to describe for you now is an example of how fantasy can free your spirit.

RECOVERY SESSION TWELVE

Guided Fantasy Adventure

You can memorize this recovery session and guide yourself through it without any help, have a friend read it to you, or use a cassette version as a guide. You can do this guided fantasy adventure literally hundreds of times and always have a unique experience, as your imagination combines with your particular feelings and mood at the time to create a unique journey. Such a session can also help reduce the need for pain medications. Of course, this session is equally helpful if you are at home in bed—your healthier friends will probably enjoy it as well!

Close your eyes when you want to. Watch your breathing. Let it be free to come and go as it wants to.

Feel your body on the bed, yawn a little perhaps. Stretch if there is tension in your muscles. And now just relax completely.

Imagine now that you are out walking, on a sunny day. You are alone, and feeling relaxed and content with the beauty of nature around you. The sun is warm, the air is clean and refreshing as you breathe.

In front of you, you see a small lake, with calm blue water, and green grass around its edges. You walk down to the edge of the water. Ducks swim in the distance.

There is a small rowboat by the water. You take off your shoes, wade to the boat, and get in. You look around and see that there is no one anywhere in sight; you are all alone to do what you want to.

So you row the boat across the lake. Enjoy the feeling in your muscles as you row. Take off your shirt if you want, feel the warmth of the sun.

You come to the middle of the lake and stop rowing. Lean back and relax completely. The sky is so blue. A few white clouds move slowly by overhead.

A gentle breeze is blowing, and you let it slowly blow your boat toward the far shore. You hear birds singing and the sound of water lapping gently against your boat. With the warmth of the sun on your skin, the breeze caressing your face, your mind drifts into memories and images that come effortlessly.

Suddenly your boat bumps gently against the shore, and awakens you. You look around and see the green grass and hillside. For a moment you don't move at all, you are so content.

Then a new energy comes in your body. You feel like walking along the road you can see nearby. So you get out of the boat, put on your shoes, and start walking along the country dirt road.

There is a strong energy in your legs. You find yourself humming a tune, perhaps whistling or singing, to express your happiness with the moment. The countryside is calm; you see animals sometimes; but there are no people out this far from town. Everyone else is busy working, but you are free, on vacation, doing what you want.

You feel so much energy in your body now that you start running a little, feeling light, almost floating along the road, powerful and graceful as you run.

The road comes to a hill. You slow down to a walk again, your legs still powerful, enjoying the climb up the hill, through trees. Birds are singing; a breeze ripples the leaves and the grass.

Your heart beats strongly as you come to the top of the hill. Suddenly, you can see over the hill into the distance. You pause to gaze at the sunset that is spreading across the sky in front of you. The colors are vibrant, so beautiful you can almost breathe the colors inside you.

Finally you start on down the other side of the hill. The road is smooth, so you start running again, feeling so light you can almost float. You flap your arms like a bird, and suddenly you are flying, effortlessly, weightless, rising above the ground, higher now, over the tops of the trees.

The feeling of flying is beautiful. You look down at the countryside below you, a breeze on your face as you fly weightless over the countryside, wherever you want to go.

Finally you choose a place to land and swoop down for a graceful landing. Your feet touch ground again. Your body feels good to be back to earth. You walk along, wondering if you really flew just then, or if it was just your vivid imagination.

Ahead, you see your house, any house you choose. You walk toward it eagerly. You can hear people's voices inside. A small party is going on. You walk into your house, your friends greet you eagerly and ask how your walk was.

A great feast has been prepared. You sit down with your friends and enjoy the wonderful food and drink in front of you. Everyone around you is so pleased with eating that there is silence except for music playing quietly in another room.

Glasses are refilled; talking begins. Someone is telling a story that strikes you as very funny. You try to hold back your laughter, but soon you are laughing without control, and everyone joins you in laughing.

Dessert comes, delicious dessert. Finally you are full. You sit talking afterward for a while as your dinner digests, drinking what you choose.

Someone puts on dance music. You feel the beat growing in your body. You want to get up and dance.

The music is your favorite dance music. Your body feels powerful and graceful as you dance around the floor with a special friend. Your other friends smile to you, and clap hands with the music.

Finally everyone is finished dancing. You sit quietly around the fireplace, watching the flames and letting your minds wander.

Then it is bedtime. Some of your guests leave to go home, some go to their guest rooms in your house, and you go up to your bedroom.

You run bathwater, and take off your clothes, enjoying the feeling of being at the end of a beautiful day. You get into the bath, and relax completely in the water, as your mind wanders where it will.

Then you get out and dry your skin slowly with a towel, noticing how good your skin feels all over. Then you go into your bedroom, and slip under the covers.

Notice if there is someone in bed with you, or if you are alone. And see what happens now!

Finally you are completely relaxed and satisfied with the day. You close your eyes, and begin to drift off into sleep.

·

Dreams come. Great wild beautiful dreams, that sweep you away into their magic spell.

And now, when you are ready, you can bring this fantasy adventure to an end, and open your eyes when you want to.

○

This guided fantasy is obviously intended to give you a beautiful experience, and some relief from the usual hospital routine. In contrast with the earlier recovery sessions, it is really aimed primarily at giving you an enjoyable vacation from the process of consciously activating your immune system. There are times when it is wonderful just to put everything aside and indulge in such fantasies. What we always seek is a balance, this time between the conscious responsible action of self-healing, and the equally important times when responsibility is put aside and pure enjoyment is called for.

So I hope that you let yourself indulge regularly in such fantasy adventures.

Recovery Tales

Have you ever healed yourself in the past? Were you ever successful, with or without the help of a doctor, in completely regaining your normal health and vitality, after falling ill or being injured?

Of course, we have all healed ourselves, many times. In fact, the healing process is constantly happening inside everyone's bodies. There are always dangerous bacteria and virus invasions roaming around our environments, entering our bodies and looking for a chance to take hold of us.

But constantly, our immune system's forces are working to identify such invaders, to surround them, and to eliminate them from our systems before they can do any harm.

And when an infection does gain dominance inside us, our immune system works overtime to generate healing and recovery.

Many people, however, have a self-image of impotence when it comes to self-healing. As children, their attitude toward sickness and recovery was conditioned so as to make them feel helpless victims, dependent upon the doctor who had to come to make them well again.

In this section of "recovery tales" I want to reinforce your self-image as a self-healer. To do this, you are once again going to turn to your memory and explore your past experiences of healing yourself. You can either simply set aside time to remember these old illnesses and injuries from which you recovered. Or you can also tell a friend about these experiences, to reinforce more strongly the process of remembering your self-healing histories. Or you can write down your "Recovery Tales." Writing can sometimes be the most powerful tool for reinforcing a memory, thus strengthening your self-image in positive directions.

The first step in this Recovery Tales process is to spend some time remembering a person who had a strong influence on you in childhood, someone related to illness and the healing process. Most of us had a memorable teacher in the early years, someone who touched us deeply with his or her wisdom. Consciously to remember this influence can be very rewarding. Or, perhaps you were influenced by someone with a very negative attitude toward "self-healing." It would also be good to remember this influence, so you can separate yourself from such attitudes.

So to begin with, give yourself time to look back into your childhood, to see where your attitudes toward self-healing come from.

Second, open yourself to remembering times in your childhood when you fell ill or somehow injured yourself. Remember the whole story, as if you are reliving each moment from beginning to end, so that you fully acknowledge the fact that you did heal yourself.

Don't bother about order—just let the memories rise to the surface as they want to. And if at first the memories are hazy, that is fine. Keep returning to them, day after day, until they become clear. Often, old illness experiences generate conditioned expectancies in your present life, undermining your self-image as a self-healer. So bring these old experiences to light and accept them, so you can be free of them.

Remember as many sickness-injury experiences as you can, and go deeply into them. You will find a vast reservoir of emotions, insights, and worthwhile experiences awaiting you!

Let me caution you again, however, not to overtax your existing personal power by pushing yourself to remember too much at once. *Remain aware of your breathing throughout, and when you feel tired, just relax your mind, do the four-word meditation to bring yourself fully back into the present moment, and return to your Recovery Tales when you feel rested.*

FINAL WORDS: LOVE AND HEALING

If you have followed this book in order, you have now learned over twenty different exercises and meditations to help you recover from illness or injury at an optimum rate. These recovery sessions, along with the Special Programs for specific chronic conditions offered in the next chapter, should provide you with a successful program for whatever your health condition might be.

As a final consideration, I should like to turn to a word, that, like *healing*, has been so overused that we sometimes tend to ignore it when talking about health and recovery. This word has to do with your relationship with the outside world, and with your self as well. It is *love*.

No scientific study has ever quantified the power of love. In fact, there is no experimental proof that love even exists. As do so many of the vital factors in health and vitality, love stands beyond the manipulative confines of the experimental method. As such, it receives no research funding; and no conferences are called to explore its function in the healing process.

Yet the healing power of love has been experienced directly by almost every one of us. Even in my journeys to Communist countries, where pragmatic materialism reigns over the scientific community, I have often found myself in late-night discussions about such factors as love in the overall picture of sickness and recovery.

The Christian tradition places utmost value on this quality of love, in all aspects of life. It goes almost without saying that hate kills, and love heals.

We find a curious biblical twist, however, when it comes to love. Jesus is quoted as saying, "Love your neighbor as you love yourself." This is quite a beautiful idea, if you happen to have an excellent love relationship with yourself. But what happens when your self-love has been eroded through negative conditioning and self-image? What happens when you do not love yourself?

Any therapist or observant doctor or nurse will give you an instant answer: some form of pain and suffering develops. And no matter how much other people who surround a sick person love this person, if there is no self-love, there is also a low incidence of recovery, especially from serious conditions such as cancer and heart disease.

So in ending this discussion on health and healing, I simply want to point in the direction of self-love. This is not a feeling that can be forced, but a feeling that can be nurtured into its own healthy glow.

We have already mentioned several of the key factors in nurturing a sense of self-love. The first is contained in the continuum between self-denial and self-acceptance. To unearth unconscious attitudes of self-rejection, to begin to consider these attitudes and to allow them to expand into a more realistic, balanced view of yourself, is a major step toward increasing self-love.

Taking one step further in this direction, we come to the realms of guilt and self-punishment for supposed past wrongs. Although the roots of the Christian tradition lie in the power of forgiveness, all too often we are conditioned into a pattern of judgment and self-condemnation, rather than acceptance and self-forgiveness. To see such habits at work in our relationship with ourselves, and to balance this attitude with the powers of compassion and acceptance, is to make another great step in the direction of self-love.

And finally, to look at your emotions, to see where they are blocked and inhibiting direct contact with the world around you, is another essential step in opening yourself to feelings of love, both for yourself and for others. Because in fact they are one and the same, the way you love yourself will always be the way you really love your neighbor.

This question of self-love is very much a matter of perceptual habits. We are talking about how you see yourself. Do you see yourself as lovable or unlovable? Once again, a preconceived attitude toward yourself will determine which aspects of yourself you do see when you look. We tend to see only what we expect to see.

I recommend that you pause regularly, perhaps four or five times a day, and consider for just a minute or two how you're feeling toward yourself. If you find you don't like yourself at that moment, say this to yourself, and watch your breathing at the same time. Notice carefully what happens to your breathing, and then to your feelings, and then to your thoughts, as you say to yourself, "I don't like myself." When you say this, a powerful process will be stimulated in your mind, as it matches this negative attitude toward yourself with recent memories and feelings—which just might run quite contrary to this attitude of self-rejection.

On the other hand, some of us carry the dominant attitude that we are really wonderful, perfect people, that we never do anything wrong, and that we are of course totally lovable. Such a totally positive attitude is just as suspect as a totally negative attitude, and can lead to as many health problems. To ignore the parts of you that would be considered "bad," to focus only on your positive traits and actions, leads to an imbalance that begins to undermine your health at unconscious levels.

To deal with this attitude habit, try saying, "Oh, I think I am really totally lovable!" and then watch your breathing, and see what happens deep down inside, as this statement is compared with usually unconscious, often contradictory, feelings toward yourself.

Love is a balance between giving and taking. Therapists who counsel ill people usually find there is an imbalance between giving and taking. Heart attack patients, for instance, are notorious for giving-giving-giving, working themselves crazy in a compulsive tendency to put out more than they get back. One way or another, this imbalance finally breaks their health. An inability to receive can be as deadly as an inability to give.

Conversely, with many cancer patients, there is a difficulty in giving, in allowing a flow of love to manifest outward to another person. There is such a hunger to receive, but the natural circular flow of love is blocked somewhere, with a resulting breakdown in connection with the outside world.

Remember that the only place such imbalances can be corrected is in the present moment. *If you find that you have an attitude of holding back your love, or of refusing love when it is offered you, then turn to the beginning pages of our discussion, and look again to your breathing for the basic lesson of giving and taking. You are continually taking the outside world into you, and then sending transformed air out into the world. Here is a constant giving and taking—and you can begin the process of opening to contact with the outside world by experiencing directly what your breathing has to teach you.*

The same is true in terms of your relationship with yourself. If you really experience your breathing, you make direct contact with "you," free of the concepts you were conditioned to apply to who you are. *If you feel your breathing coming and going without effort, and then expand to feel your heart—there you are, and there you will find a new chance to establish an honest, balanced, loving relationship with this person you call you.*

Perhaps the best next step in our discussion is for me to stop presenting new information and techniques for healing, and allow you to return to the beginning of the discussion and step by step, experiment again with the sessions. Find the ones most directly active for you, and spend your time seeing what new experiences and healing powers come to you as you explore your healing potential.

If you are suffering from one of the specific health conditions mentioned in the following pages, you will find Dr. von Lühmann's suggestions and special cure programs of great help, when combined with the more general techniques already discussed. A Bibliography of important books on the various health conditions is listed as well. Also, cassette programs that guide you through the various aspects of healing mentioned in our discussion will be outlined in case you want to turn to such professional guidance in your own home.

SPECIAL PROGRAMS

As I have mentioned several times already, the programs in this book have been strongly influenced by the insights and practical medical techniques of my colleague, Dr. Manfred von Lühmann. In this final section, I am going to present for you a number of specific cure techniques drawn from Dr. von Lühmann's innovative work.

You will find that there is a strong common link between the various programs for different health conditions in this section. In order to understand the heart of Dr. von Lühmann's approach to self-healing, I would recommend that you read through this entire section before applying the suggestions to your particular condition. Even if you do not suffer from one of these ailments, I think you will find the discussions rewarding.

Special Diets and Fasting Cures

In Chapter 7, "Proper Foods for Recovery," we began our exploration of the relationship between the food you eat and your health. Now we can go deeper into more specific suggestions.

For instance, if you suffer from gas pains and bloating, you should immediately stop or seriously reduce your intake of sugar, juices, and white flour. Do your best to eat only twice a day, in the morning and afternoon, with five hours between meals. For dinner, limit yourself to a dish of soup. Also, avoid all high-protein foods for a seven-day period, to give your intestines a chance to regain a more healthy bacterial balance.

Recent research has pointed out another important step you can take for your condition. This has to do with the ways in which you cook your food. It has been shown that cooking proteins together with carbohydrates creates complex chemical compounds in food that are very difficult for enzymes in the small intestine and stomach to separate and digest. These undigested compounds then go into the large intestine, where bacteria attack the compounds and generate gas and a fermentation-putrefication condition.

So whether you are baking, frying, or boiling your food, separate the protein foods from the carbohydrates, and you will quite probably notice positive results in your condition within a few days.

If the condition in your stomach is especially severe, don't eat these two types of food at the same time, and instead let your stomach work to digest one type at a time.

Once you have regained new health in your intestines, the important step is to develop a habit of eating live, fresh foods, of not eating after six in the evening, and of cooking your foods properly.

In Chapter 5, "Emotions and the Immune System," I stressed the importance of reducing chronic anxiety and mental worry in your life. Acidic stomachs are a reflection of tension, stress, and past-future mind states. Conscious relaxation and present-moment awareness are as essential in resolving stomach disorders as is a change in diet.

Constipation is also a function of the food you take in and the emotions in which you're caught up. I am sure you know already such basic advice as increasing your intake of roughage to reduce constipation. You will also want to reduce your intake of animal fats, which tend to clog up the large intestine if not properly digested in the stomach and small intestine. And, once again, eat live natural foods to the exclusion of refined flour and sugar products.

Regular exercise is one of the other main ingredients in developing a healthy regularity.

As can be imagined, chronic addiction to such foods as sugar, white-flour products, and heavy animal fats stands directly in the way of regaining healthy intestinal flora. These addictions are often associated with chronic tiredness, and reflect a basic imbalance of the body.

Very often, it is necessary to put yourself on a total fast to break free of habitual eating patterns that you know are bad for your health. Or if you don't want to take such an extreme step, at least make sure that you stop buying sugars and white-flour products, so they are not available in your house.

Digestion Disorders

Hand in hand with digestive problems go the various food allergies that plague so many of us. Recent research has shed increasing light on the cause of food allergies. Basically, allergies usually begin with a change in the mucous membranes of the intestines brought about by chronic unbalanced eating habits, usually dating from childhood. When the permeability of the mucous membranes is changed due to faulty eating, then wrong compounds are taken into the bloodstream.

It is at this point that allergic reactions begin. Usually

the medical treatment for allergies tries to treat the symptoms. But the heart of the problem seems to lie in the mucous membrane and the flora of the intestines themselves, rather than in the particular food being eaten.

So a deeper treatment for food allergies often begins with fasting. Through this alteration in your eating, enzymes and bacteria can regain their natural balance, and the mucous membranes lining the digestive tract regain their healthy functioning.

Another approach to food allergies is the Rotating Diet. You eat one food, rice for instance, for one day, then avoid rice for the next four days before eating it again. Thus you completely change your diet each new day, giving your intestines a rest from each particular food for at least four days. In this diet, you want to avoid animal fat and protein as much as possible, and also be sure to eat your food slowly and in a relaxed state.

Very often, food allergies seem to be intimately related to habitual anxiety patterns. In a state of chronic stress, we tend to eat our food in such a hurry that our digestive processes cannot function properly. If this is your habit, you should consciously begin to alter it toward more relaxed eating. For instance: pause for eight breaths of silence before eating your first bite; and take a breath in between each subsequent bite. Let your mind come into the present moment by focusing on perceptions rather than thoughts; and relax the muscles of your body.

Also, avoid fruit and sugar products that tend to stimulate you into manic behavior. Don't eat after five or six in the evening when possible. And try giving yourself three or four periods of at least five minutes a day when you have absolutely nothing to do but relax and watch the world go by!

There is a remarkable test, called the Pulse Test, that you can give yourself to determine which foods are causing allergic reactions of tiredness, irritation, stomach problems, and so forth. The Pulse Test, which is very accurate, is based on the fact that your pulse rate will increase by at least eight beats a minute from normal within half an hour after eating something to which you are allergic.

First, measure your pulse for three days on waking and just before falling asleep, to find your normal pulse rate. Measure your pulse by placing three fingertips on the thumb side of your wrist, palm up, for one minute.

Once you have determined your normal resting pulse, measure it just before eating (after having rested for perhaps three to five minutes) to see if your pulse rate matches your normal rate.

Now go ahead and eat your meal; and then half an hour after the meal, measure your pulse again. If it is eight or more beats higher than before the meal, and you haven't been exercising to increase your pulse, then you know that you ate something to which you are allergic.

At this point, you will want to have a meal of nothing but the food you suspect you are allergic to, to see if your pulse goes up again. Once you have identified the food you are allergic to, avoid this food for four weeks, then add it to the Rotating Diet (eat it every four days) to see if your allergy has disappeared.

TOOTH INFECTIONS. Many of us, even without knowing it, suffer from chronic tooth infections that poison our bloodstream and tax our immune systems. Acidic saliva further aggravates this condition. Proper treatment involves change in diet and emotional habits. The main cause of hyperacidity in the mouth comes from daily intake of white-flour foods and sugar products. Usually such a diet is low in raw and fresh vegetables and whole grains. So see if you can reverse this balance in favor of live foods.

Emotions such as anger and anxiety also generate an acidic saliva content. Chronic tense tongue and jaw muscles add to this condition. So you might want to return at some point to such chapters as 3 and 5 on how consciously to deal with emotional and physical tensions.

There is serious concern among medical professionals regarding the use of amalgam (dark metal) fillings. These fillings are inexpensive compared with gold or plastic and are commonly used. But they happen to contain serious amounts of mercury, which poisons the system at subtle levels.

Many symptoms related to this mercury poisoning are now suspected, including allergies, intestinal problems, rashes, and nervousness. If you are in excellent health, your body can probably deal with the mercury adequately. But when your health is not good, then this toxic amalgam in your mouth can be another factor that pulls you down and keeps you from regaining your health. This, along with possible chronic infections under your fillings, makes your teeth an important consideration if recovery eludes you.

Although Manfred usually recommends avoiding X-ray exposure, he suggests here that you might consider having your teeth x-rayed if your health seems somehow under chronic stress. Find out for sure if you have any infected roots under your fillings, and if you do, go to the expense and pain of having the root removed.

Chinese acupuncture links each tooth root with a particular organ or region in the body. As long as the tooth infection continues, the organ difficulty remains. Possibly, if you deal with the tooth infection, you will find other health problems much improved as a result, because your immune system will be free of its constant fight against the tooth infection, and will have power to put its resources elsewhere as needed.

CHRONIC INFECTIONS. Besides tooth infections, we should mention chronic sinus troubles, tonsil problems, bladder and kidney infections, and chronic appendix difficulties as well. These lymphatic infections are also directly linked with improper eating habits that upset the basic mucous membrane functioning of the intestines and interfere with the natural processing of food into energy compounds in the bloodstream.

Along with the advice mentioned already for chronic infections, Manfred recommends a high intake of green leafy foods such as salads and spinach. A diet high in chlorophyll will alter the breathing potential of certain bacteria that need to be reduced in numbers, and thus will improve the balance in the intestines rapidly. If you have access to wheat-grass juice, you will find this the most powerful way to take in chlorophyll. You simply buy wheat-grass seeds at any health-food store, sprout them in a small amount of soil, and eight days after planting, you have grass to cut and put through the juicer. Drinking an ounce a day, mixed with tomato juice, is highly recommended.

Antibiotics are often given for chronic infections and they do succeed in killing off some of the infectious bacteria in the body. But because antibiotics do not change the terrain, the environment inside the intestines, the bacteria can return. This is why, for a genuine cure from an infection, you need to alter your diet, to change the environment in which the bacteria grow. Only with this deep change can you truly overcome infection problems.

Hypoglycemia

In strict medical terms, hypoglycemia, an abnormal decrease of sugar in the blood, is caused by overstimulation of the insulin-producing organ, the pancreas. It is estimated that over 25 percent of us suffer from this chronic condition, even though we might not have been diagnosed as such.

The symptoms include sudden bouts of shakiness,

rapid pulse, tight breathing, a craving for sweets or alcohol or other drugs, and then exhaustion. In extreme cases, a severe headache accompanies these symptoms, followed by vomiting.

The symptoms almost exactly parallel those of chronic anxiety patients. We have all felt the symptoms at times, when stress and anxiety have thrown our organs off balance and upset our blood-sugar levels. But many people have this as a regular daily condition, and it is really a terrible chronic experience.

There is much argument about the causes of hypoglycemia. Biochemists are trying to prove that it is a simple malfunctioning of the body, to be treated with chemicals. Psychologists tend to insist that the source of the condition is at least partly emotional, stemming from childhood emotional conditioning related to fear of one kind or another. It is very often associated with people who are running compulsively after goals, afraid of failure, and not reflecting on what they would really want to do in life. In these people a conflict persists between the "should" of survival behavior, and the deeper emotional needs of the person.

Hypoglycemic people tend to leave themselves no free time to relax and enjoy themselves. They always keep themselves busy, busy, busy, stimulating their anxiety feelings by worrying about the future, and somehow running away from something deep in the past.

Certainly, the basic dietary wisdom thus far in our discussion applies directly to hypoglycemia as well. Cut the sugars and white-flour foods as much as possible, eat live fresh foods, and avoid heavy animal fats.

But also pause and take a look at your living habits. See what you are doing to yourself. Notice if you are treating yourself in a way that you enjoy, or if you push yourself so that there is no pleasure in life.

The basic rule for the hypoglycemic is: Face your danger. Turn and look at what you are running from all the time. Take a deep breath and come into the present moment; let yourself relax.

These are easy words to say, but often almost impossible to attain unless you start right at the heart of the matter: your breathing. If you are in a chronic state of excitement and anticipation, pushing into the future with fear breathing down your neck from behind, then your breathing will be uptight, shallow, and lack a good relaxed exhale.

You can set free your breathing—we have discussed how throughout this book. And if shakiness, sudden anxiety, tiredness, and sweets addiction are problems for you, you will want to return to our chapters on emotional growth, especially Chapter 5, as you also begin to alter your diet in positive directions. And, of course, at times the help of a therapist can stimulate rapid growth.

Diabetes

Diabetes is caused when the insulin-producing cells in the pancreas become exhausted and stop making insulin. When this happens, the blood sugar is no longer broken down for fuel for the cells of the body, and a serious condition of coma and resultant death can ensue within hours.

Luckily, we live in an age when insulin can be injected to replace the loss of an organic inner supply, so diabetes is a condition with which one can live a full lifetime.

It should be made clear that hypoglycemia, in which the pancreas gland is overstimulated, is often the first stage of diabetes, in which the gland finally gives out through chronic overwork. In fact, diabetes is properly called *hyper* (as opposed to hypo)*glycemia,* to show this direct relationship.

The first symptoms of a failure of the pancreas gland are a dry mouth, thirst after eating, and a craving for sweets. Frequent urination, loss of weight, and reduction in energy and mental clarity accompany a gradual failure of the pancreatic production of insulin. If you have these symptoms, you should speak with your doctor about taking a test to determine the functioning of your pancreas.

However, we must also place prediabetic symptoms within the emotional realms of the body, because there is a strong link between certain emotional/mental states and a tendency to develop diabetes, especially after the age of thirty-five. Chronic anxiety, worrying, and stress do stimulate the pancreas, especially when one's diet is high in sugar and white-flour products.

Prediabetic people can act consciously to reduce their chronic stress habits. Thus they can reduce the strain on the pancreas gland—and sometimes overcome the symptoms of prediabetes, saving themselves from having to develop a defective pancreas condition. Much of our program in this book can be directly applied to such a reversal in one's emotional and life-style patterns.

I should mention before going any further that there are two distinct types of diabetes: childhood, or primary, diabetes, and onset diabetes. Childhood diabetes seems to have a strong genetic component, along with a particular immune reaction to one's own insulin. No one yet knows why this immune reaction happens, but it has been found that sometimes treatment with an immune-modulation technique, in which desensitization is gained through ingestion of cellular material extracted from the thymus gland, can help a child overcome this pancreas failure.

If you have a family history of diabetes and are a parent, you will want to help your child avoid sugar and white-flour foods. Total avoidance is usually not a wise policy, though, because this can generate emotional reactions that backfire at a later date.

You will also want to consider whether your family seems to pass from generation to generation certain emotional patterns that place stress on the pancreas gland and thus push a child into a diabetic condition. It has been found that diabetic personalities tend to be nice, quiet, obedient people, blocking emotional expression, especially the appropriate discharge of anger. Guilt tends to be associated with pleasure, and a general inhibition mixed with anxiety.

This inhibition/anxiety/stress profile will generate stress and tensions in the body, stimulating an overproduction of insulin to match the stress state in the body/emotions. There is not enough relaxation, not enough fun, not enough free time, not enough acceptance of the natural human emotions and needs. Focus in such families is on achievement, morality, survival fears, and social standing. If the pancreas gland is somewhat weak through genetics, then the additional emotional stress will cause the gland to burn out; had the emotional stress not been present in childhood, the gland might have continued throughout life.

Please do not think that I am placing blame on parents for children who develop diabetes. We all do the best we can, given our genetic/emotional/social inheritance, and we are just beginning to understand the relationship between emotions and physical disease. So please don't even consider guilt; but feel instead the challenge of doing all you can to gain new information to take care of your children and yourself at the pancreatic level.

Most important is the encouragement of emotional expression and the discharge of pleasure and anger, sad feelings and bright feelings. The homes of diabetic families all too often offer no release valves for emotional expression: everything from breathing to verbalization is inhibited. The best path out of this inhibition/stress condition is to begin simply with breathing, movement, honest observation, and communication.

The second type of diabetes, which usually strikes people over the age of forty, seems to be much more emotional than genetic in its development. There must be a genetic predisposition for a weak pancreas for diabetes to develop. But the emotional profile of the person will determine how soon, and how severely, a pancreas malfunction will occur.

Even if you have already developed diabetes, there is much you can do for yourself at the emotional level, to help with your physical condition. You can do as your doctor has already told you: avoid sugar, white-flour products, and alcohol. Eat regularly and not too much at a time. It is strongly advised that *all* caffeine products, including coffee, cola, and nonherbal teas, be eliminated completely from your diet.

Instead give your pancreas wonderful food, relaxed days, and let your heart open so that there is more of a loving flow between you and the outside world. To reduce anxiety at a deep level, you will want to take a good look at your mortality, at the reality that you are going to die someday. Chronic anxiety is pointless. Worrying about tomorrow is foolish when you could be enjoying the present moment!

Cancer

Like the other conditions we are discussing in this section, cancer is a complex condition that continues to elude medical comprehension. However, with each passing week and month, we gain deeper insights into the nature of the disease, and thus we can offer practical suggestions that may help you if you are struggling with cancer in one form or another.

Dr. von Lühmann focuses on six levels of treatment for cancer at his own clinic for cancer recovery in Kassel. These six levels are: detoxification medications; proper diet; reduced infections (teeth, and so forth); special movement programs; emotional disinhibition; and attitudinal transformation.

The deeper new understanding of cancer focuses on the relationship between consciousness and cancer cells. Recent research has shown that we simply cannot separate mind from body, that the two function together as a biochemical-electrical whole. At the level of acupuncture and meridian energy flows throughout the body, there even seems to be a more subtle energy relationship among the mind, emotions, and cellular functioning.

Cancer cells seem to be suffering from isolation from a positive flow of both energy (bioelectrical) and metabolism. People with cancer tend to have pulled their consciousness away from the region of the body that develops the cancerous growth. This loss of body consciousness very possibly lies at the core of the cause of cancer—and also the cure. For this reason, I have devoted Chapter 4 of this book to the healing process of Direct Focusing, which you have already read.

When the mind pulls away from a region of the body, it is usually part of a more general avoidance pattern. The region of the body being ignored is somehow linked emotionally with an unbearable pain or fear. In order to escape from confrontation with this core fear or pain, the mind unconsciously withdraws basic dynamic awareness from this region. The result is a malfunctioning of the cells, and a regression back to an embryonic functioning that results in proliferation of the cancerous tissue.

As an added piece of the cancer puzzle, let me mention that people with low anxiety and high love/acceptance personality profiles do not tend to get cancer, but people of the opposite profile—high anxiety, low love/acceptance profiles—are especially prone to cancer.

What positive suggestions can be made to reverse the cancer condition? As we have already discussed, correct diet is of great value in freeing the body's metabolism for maximum immune-system functioning. Dealing with chronic infections such as those in the roots of the teeth is another positive step you can make. Movement programs such as yoga, and the special movement/personal power programs outlined already are important as well. Emotional release, as discussed previously, is essential. And the detoxification programs such as developed by Dr. von Lühmann further the possibility of genuine recovery.

But there is also the underlying question of your attitude toward yourself. Do you really accept yourself? Can you be honest about the parts of yourself that you deny, that you reject (especially in terms of past experiences you have had, things you have done)? And can you look directly at your feelings of love for yourself, and begin to open your heart once again to a positive flow of feelings?

Reconnection with positive attitudes is at the heart of cancer recovery. What are your attitudes toward life in general? Are they positive or negative? Do you love being alive, or not?

And what really is the source of all the anxiety you may feel inside you? What are you afraid of deep down? What are you trying to kill off inside you?

If in fact you are suffering from cancer, I can only suggest that you return to the beginning of our discussion, and step by step, go through the various chapters a number of times. See where you feel the urge to skip over a chapter or paragraph. See where you reject what I am saying. See what excuses you create to avoid doing the healing sessions.

In short, get to know yourself better, using this discussion as a mirror to your old attitudes. And instead of judging yourself for negative attitudes—accept yourself. We are all of us imperfect, struggling souls; and our only hope in evolving is to accept ourselves as we are.

Heart Disease

There is, deep down, quite a similarity between cancer and heart disease, because we find that heart attack patients also suffer from an inhibition in the flow of basic emotions through the body, and from a denial of certain aspects of themselves. Certain personality qualities are almost always lacking in heart attack patients. Let me first of all give you a list of qualities that are found in people who almost never have heart attacks:

1. People who can sit quietly at peace, and listen to the silence around them, and be in harmony with their surroundings, almost never end up in the hospital with heart problems.

2. People who are satisfied with their life, who have a calm sense of acceptance of the flow of life day to day, are also free of heart attacks.

3. People who remain in touch with the feelings they had naturally as little children, are especially free of heart difficulties.

4. People who have open hearts, who can give away their flow of emotion freely to others, and make contact deeply at the emotional level, are never bothered with heart disease.

Am I describing you?

We used to blame stress for causing heart attacks. But it is now well documented that many high-pressured executives under extreme stress from their work have beautifully healthy hearts. As long as their hearts are open and there is a feeling of full participation in life and full acceptance of the flow of life, an appreciation of the fun of life, then stress doesn't kill.

We also often blame diet for causing heart attacks, especially high animal fat diets. But the traditional Eskimos who live on an unbelievably high-fat diet have almost no incidence of heart disease.

Only when we combine stress and diet with other factors do we gain a clear picture of what leads to heart disease. So now let us look at the personality qualities that do seem almost always to be present in heart-attack patients:

1. Fighting against the clock, struggling against the system, battling against fate—these attitudes are linked intimately with heart disease. When one's sense of time is thrown off, when one is pushing constantly into the future instead of living directly in the present moment, then stress becomes negative. Ambition is certainly a deadly personality quality, because it always is accompanied by an underlying fear profile that pushes the person constantly against the natural flow of time and life.

2. Chronic activity, inability to relax and enjoy the present moment—again, fear of pausing and accepting the natural rhythms of life—almost always accompany heart problems. Children know how to play, how to be totally in the present moment, and to enjoy each eternal experience as it comes to them. Many adults lose this ability and lose touch with their inner child—and push themselves in directions with which the inner child cannot live.

3. We come here to the essence of heart disease—a violation of the inner child's needs. Much talk has been offered in recent years concerning the American Indian's notion of the "heart path," in which one moves through life choosing to go in directions that make the heart feel good and whole and in harmony with all of life. When this heart path is violated, over a period of time, through decisions that choose ambition (fear) over participation (love), then the inner child begins to wither, the heart grows hard, and great conflict exists within the heart region.

Just as cancer is a withdrawal of loving attention from a region of the body, so is heart disease a withdrawal of loving attention specifically from the region of the heart. In simple terms, when you break your "child's heart" step by ambitious step, you reach a point where the pain in your heart becomes a physiological spasm—the pain of an isolated heart becomes manifest, and down you go.

It is hoped that your first heart attack does not kill you and you come out of the hospital with a changed heart. You will have learned a giant lesson, which you now must try to apply. This is perhaps the most important step of your life. Can you change your manic, ambitious pace in life? Have you learned that there is more to life than success and dominance? Have you found that you can face what scares you deep down, and let go of the anxieties that seem to push you forward so compulsively? And have you found that there is a little boy or girl alive and well inside you, with whom you can now reestablish a loving, playful relationship?

In sum: change your diet to healthy natural foods; enjoy the present moment; experience every new breath you take; risk opening your heart and letting people around you feel your true, uninhibited emotional flow; live today and let tomorrow take care of itself when it comes; get out in nature as much as possible; work up a sweat every day doing good, worthwhile work; and every day, include love with a big dash of acceptance in your diet.

Give your feelings away for free.

The AIDS Question

Because dedicated AIDS experts who have been working night and day for years admit that they have very little deep understanding of the nature of the AIDS epidemic, it would be naïve of me to pretend that I can offer a few golden words to clarify this worldwide health problem.

What I want to do instead is to focus our general discussion onto the AIDS question. We do know that the human immunodeficiency virus (HIV) is the prime cause of the disease, and we do know that AIDS symptoms develop directly as a result of various immune-system dysfunctions in the body of an infected person. What we don't yet know is this: Why do many people who are tested to be AIDS-positive postpone developing the deadly symptoms, even though they are contaminated by the virus, while a relatively small percentage of those infected quickly fall victim to the terrible deterioration of health that happens when the virus succeeds in undermining the functioning of the immune system?

It is always a foolish thing to try to find one solitary cause of any health problem. Life is not so simple as experimental models would imply. And I feel that there are a number of variables that contribute to an AIDS-positive person's fate.

Variables we cannot alter very much include the genetic strengths and weaknesses of our bodily system, which certainly contribute to the ability of the infected person's system to fight off the virus. Another variable we can do little to affect is the factor of simple fate, of chance probability of the virus happening to be lucky in its attack on the immune system of a person. Life for all of us is constantly affected by genetic endowment and chance, and we must simply roll with the punches and accept this level of our lives with as open and positive an attitude as possible.

But the other two main variables that seem to influence strength or weakness in fighting off AIDS symptoms are in fact at least somewhat within our personal control. We have been talking about these variables all through this book: living habits and attitudes.

A great deal has already been written in the last few years concerning the negative dimensions of life-style of most drug addicts, and of many gay people as well. From my experience, some descriptions of these life-styles have been realistic, while other descriptions have been overly negative. If you fall into one of these categories and are also AIDS-positive, you can judge for yourself if your habitual life-style lends itself to the healthy qualities of life we have been discussing, or if in fact there is an underlying antilife and antihealth structure to your everyday routines.

Coupled intimately with the life-style question is of course the question of your chronic thought patterns, emotional habits, and attitudes. These inner personality qualities you have developed all your life can be an active force in pulling you down deeper into a death spiral. And I know that such habits are difficult to change. But if you have found out that you are AIDS-positive, then you will certainly be strongly motivated to transform your life where needed, if you do in fact want to prolong your life.

And here we confront again the issue of death. We all die sometime. Who is to say when the right time to die has come in each of our lives?

My basic suggestion is this: do your best to look deeply inside yourself. Don't just blindly react to the fear of dying. Take a look at death itself. This is an ultimate challenge. If you are AIDS-positive, you are in the same position as Carlos Castaneda's archetypal warrior—you have death constantly over your left shoulder, to serve you as either best friend and counselor or to push you into the state of anxiety and contraction that makes you ideal ground for an immune-system breakdown.

I also suggest that you seek out both professional and lay help in your journey to the heart of the life-death question. Find someone who is willing to be honest with you, who doesn't treat you like a helpless victim. Find someone who can serve as a fellow explorer into this ultimate of questions.

·

In terms of specific programs for keeping your immune system as strong as possible, I suggest that you go back over the programs already outlined in this book, and find the ones that seem most powerful for you. By adding one, two, or three of these primary meditations to your daily routine, you will find that you have acted to stimulate transformation. Yours is an ultimate challenge, and this is why I am not mincing words at this point. I do not know the whole picture of AIDS, and all I can offer you are the techniques we have discussed, which have proved most effective. I hope that they prove to be a lifeline for you, so you can contact the special spirit within you that will keep you from falling into AIDS symptoms.

For those of you who have already developed AIDS symptoms, I do not pretend to hold out any miracle cures for you as you face an extremely difficult life situation. At the same time, I do want to say that miracles do happen, and I hope that you can find some of the meditations in this book helpful to your moment-to-moment experiences, whatever they may be. My first instinct is to tell you that there is hope, that you should take this book of immune-system activation techniques and make it your bible, devoting yourself to seeing what you can in fact do to fight against the virus that has you in its grip. But at the same time, having had friends who have died from AIDS, I know that it is as important to face death clearly and positively as it is to keep up the fight to live. So I suggest that you do this: take whatever guilt you still carry around, and dump it once and for all out of your life. And then use that extra energy that comes into you when you let go of guilt feelings to spur your immune system into heroic action.

One of the most debilitating factors AIDS patients have to struggle against is the attitude of people around them who see them as helpless victims, whose attitude pushes them even further into difficult states. You cannot act to help yourself as long as you see yourself as a help-less victim.

I would like also to address the question of personal responsibility. It does no good to carry around the attitude that you are not responsible for what happens inside your body. Certainly you are as responsible as you are capable of being. Even if it was pure chance that AIDS got into your bloodstream, from here on out you can take responsi-bility for what happens inside you. Deal with the past realistically, without guilt. Most important, fight back against the people around you who are laying the "help-less victim" routine on you all the time. Tell them that you want to be seen as someone who takes responsibility for him- or herself in the present moment. Tell them you want your integrity back, and your freedom to ride this AIDS current wherever it takes you, without being stripped of your basic sense of self-determination. And if you are dying, then insist on a deep and meaningful experience while you are still alive, and as you pass on to the other side.

There often comes a time when the person who is sick must take the affirmative action with those around him or her. You need to help your friends and medical support team to grow until they are not afraid to talk honestly with you. It is only when you confront them about their inhibitions that they can open up and offer you the support that you need, in order to reach a deeper level of consciousness.

When this transformation comes to you, when you find that you can look at yourself honestly, face death straight-on, and feel in charge of your own fate, no matter what it may be, then I feel that in fact, miracles are possi-ble. If it is your fate to be one of the first to tell the AIDS virus to get lost, then power to you. If not, love and an infinite beyond to you!

I should perhaps say a word about AIDS as it relates to those of us who have not—at least as yet—contracted the virus in our bloodstream. At the present moment, as I am sure you know, the dominant medical opinion is that the only ways you can become infected with the virus are through blood contamination, sexual contact, and birth from an infected mother.

This means two things. First, you can be with someone who is AIDS-positive or suffering from AIDS symptoms without fear of getting the disease yourself, as long as you avoid relating in the particular ways that can spread the disease. Second, you can carry on with your normal life without becoming overly paranoid in your sexual relationships.

I think it is important that we stay conscious of paranoid tendencies both within ourselves, and within our culture as a whole, when it comes to the AIDS question. Certainly there is the possibility that the AIDS virus can somehow mutate and spread to the general population. There is even the chance that a large part of the population could be wiped out by the disease, as in fact happened with the plague in the Middle Ages. Terrible disasters do befall civilizations from time to time.

But a proper perspective can help us to face even terrible times. Let us face our coming death, be it next week or in fifty years, with the respect and bravery necessary to transform the ultimate human demise into the ultimate human fulfillment. It is not a coincidence that I end a book on how to heal yourself by talking about how to die with respect and an inner sense of balance and readiness.

My suspicion is that those people who are best able to heal themselves are exactly those who have looked death in the eye and accepted its reality alongside the reality of life. When your fear of death drops to a lower intensity within you, you have more available energy for encouraging the healing process within you. So we can take heart in a paradox: when we accept that we are going to die, we are able to live more fully.

Since we will all die someday, we all have the opportunity to see this reality of life, and to make the most of the valuable and limited time we have left on this planet.

In this light, the AIDS epidemic presents a powerful challenge, the limits of which we still have not guessed. Our response to this challenge will determine a great deal, I suspect, about the fate of human beings on this planet of ours. Perhaps we will finally realize that we are one world, like it or not, and that our fate rests at least partially in our conscious ability to take responsibility for our own health, and to work to improve our human equilibrium. The balance between life and death, between survival and extinction, between sickness and health, does somehow rest in the hands of each of us. And it seems that the only way to affect that balance in a positive manner is to come directly into the present moment where growth is possible, and see what we can do with our own personal lives to encourage inner balance, health, and love.

SUPPORTING
PROGRAMS

PROFESSIONAL CASSETTE TAPES

There are times when it is very helpful to be able to put down the written descriptions of the various programs described in this book and listen to a professional voice that guides you through the healing sessions. Such guidance can take you very deeply into the particular states of mind that you need to stimulate the healing process.

The following cassette programs have been developed by me and my partner, Birgitta Steiner, to give you gentle but powerful guidance to the heart of the sessions you find most effective for your particular needs. Each session lasts about twenty minutes, with additional music to round off the session.

Immune-System Activation Cassette One

SIDE A: REGAINING THE PRESENT MOMENT. This primary healing meditation, which you have learned in the book, becomes especially powerful when a guiding voice takes responsibility for the structure of the meditation, and you are free to expand your awareness deeply into the healing vitality of the ongoing present moment. The program in the book has been expanded in this guided recovery session to include important dimensions of several other of the healing sessions as well.

SIDE B: HEALING-MOVEMENT PROGRAM. This recovery session guides you through the different gentle movements which you have been introduced to in the book, and serves strongly to stimulate your general level of vitality. If you are physically unable to do the movements, you can follow the suggestions in your imagination, and actually experience changes in your physiological functioning through this fantasy experiencing of the movements.

Immune-System Activation Cassette Two

SIDE A: HAND-DIRECTED INTEGRATION (ENERGY BALANCING). This cassette is dedicated to the use of your hands for stimulating a flow of healing energy throughout your body. On side A, you are guided gently through the hand integration recovery session, where you focus your attention on the different energy centers under your hands and quickly generate an integrated and balanced relationship between the different centers in your body. The session has been expanded to include a healing meditation toward the end as well.

SIDE B: HEALING THROUGH DIRECT FOCUSING. You can do this recovery session either on its own, or directly following side A as a longer experience. In this session you relax and expand your awareness to your whole body, and then turn your attention directly to that part of your body that needs a special influx of healing attention. You also use your hands to enhance the healing process and employ several verbal meditations to bring your entire being into focus for stimulating the healing process.

Immune-System Activation Cassette Three

SIDE A: EMOTIONAL BALANCING. As you learned in the text, there is a simple yet very powerful technique for balancing your various emotions. You will be effortlessly guided through the twelve emotional states in this recovery session, so that you feel balanced and full of the life-force that lies at the heart of your feelings.

SIDE B: RELEASE AND HEALING OF EMOTIONS. This recovery session first gives you guidance in releasing pent-up emotions, and then leads you into a relaxed open emotional state that provides the perfect take-off point for a deep healing meditation.

Immune-System Activation Cassette Four

SIDE A: MEMORY HEALING. A guiding voice is especially powerful in helping you to go back into various dimensions of your past, to relive experiences, to let go of old contractions, and to regain the vitality of your youthful spirit. This recovery session ends with a special meditation that brings you back into the present moment while enabling you to retain the healing vitality you have encountered in the session.

SIDE B: FREE FANTASY ADVENTURES. This recovery session is pure enjoyment, guiding you into beautiful fantasies that will let your spirit soar while your body relaxes and opens to the healing process. It is important to give yourself such times of escape and pleasure while you are sick, and even after you have recovered.

Immune-System Activation Cassette Five

"ZEN TUNES": SPECIAL MUSIC FOR HEALING.   This collection of music has been composed and recorded to stimulate deep relaxation and peace both in the mind and in the body. Drawing from both classical, Oriental, and gentle jazz influences, the music gives you space to meditate upon the healing process, rather than pulling your attention to the music itself. With a great variety of instruments and themes, the music should offer a lifetime of meditative enjoyment.

To order any of these cassette programs, please write to John Selby Programs, P.O. Box 8320, Santa Fe, NM 87504.
Individual cassettes: $12.00 (includes postage).
Complete set of 5 cassettes: $48.00 (check or money order). (We will process your order and mail you your cassettes within five days, with satisfaction guaranteed.)

TRAINING/HEALING SEMINARS

Along with the book and cassette programs, we also offer regular weekend and extended seminars to take you deeper into the various healing programs described in the text, and also to present additional techniques presently being perfected by me and my staff. The full program offered monthly in Santa Barbara includes thirty hours of instruction and healing sessions. Room and board are available for those of you from out of town. Please write for further information and reservations to Mauritzia Zannin at the Santa Fe address above.

We also offer periodic professional training programs for doctors, nurses, therapists, ministers, and other interested health practitioners who would like credential instruction in the programs outlined in this book. For information on such training seminars, please write as well to the above address. And if you would like to arrange for a healing seminar to be offered in your region, also contact Mauritzia in Santa Fe. We hope that these various cassette programs and seminars serve your personal needs as you act to enhance your healing potential!

BIBLIOGRAPHY

ADER, ROBERT, ed. *Psychoneuroimmunology.* New York: Academic Press, 1981.

ALEXANDER, FRANZ. *Psychosomatic Medicine.* New York: Norton, 1965.

BENSON, HERBERT. *The Mind-Body Effect.* New York: Berkley, 1980.

———. *The Relaxation Response.* New York: Morrow, 1975.

BESOLWITZ, B. L. *Anxiety and Stress.* New York: McGraw-Hill, 1955.

BLUM, R. *The Management of the Doctor-Patient Relationship.* New York: McGraw-Hill, 1960.

BROWN, BARBARA. *New Mind, New Body.* New York: Harper & Row, 1975.

BURTON, R. *The Anatomy of Melancholy.* New York: Tudor, 1941.

BUSCAGLIA, LEO. *Living, Loving & Learning.* New York: Fawcett, 1983.

———. *Love.* New York: Ballantine, 1982.

CANNON, W. B. *The Wisdom of the Body.* New York: Norton, 1963.

CAPRA, FRITJOF. *The Tao of Physics*. New York: Bantam Books, 1981.

CASTANEDA, CARLOS. *Tales of Power*. New York: Simon & Schuster, 1975.

CASTIGLIONE, A. *A History of Medicine*. New York: Alfred A. Knopf, 1947.

COLGROVE, MELBA. *How to Survive the Loss of a Love*. New York: Bantam Books, 1977.

COUSINS, NORMAN. *The Anatomy of an Illness*. New York: Norton, 1979.

DODGE, D. L. *Social Stress and Illness*. South Bend, Ind.: University of Notre Dame Press, 1970.

DOSSEY, LARRY. *Space, Time & Medicine*. Boulder, Colo.: Shambala, 1977.

DUBOS, RENÉ. *Health and Disease*. New York: Time/Life Books, 1965.

———. *Man, Medicine, & Environment*. New York: Praeger, 1968.

———. *Mirage of Health*. New York: Harper & Row, 1971.

DUNBAR, F. *Emotions and Bodily Changes*. New York: Columbia University Press, 1954.

EVANS, ELIDA. *A Psychological Study of Cancer*. New York: Dodd & Mead, 1926.

EVERSON, T. C. *Spontaneous Regression of Cancer*. Philadelphia: Saunders, 1966.

FOSSHAGE, JAMES. *Healing: Implications for Psychotherapy*. New York: Human Sciences Press, 1978.

GARFIELD, CHARLES, ed. *Psychosocial Care of the Dying Patient*. New York: McGraw-Hill, 1978.

GLASSMAN, JUDITH. *The Cancer Survivors: And How They Did It*. New York: Doubleday, 1983.

GOLAS, T. *The Lazy Man's Guide to Enlightenment*. New York: Bantam Books, 1972.

GUNDERSON, E. K., ed. *Life Stress and Illness*. Springfield, Ill.: Thomas Charles, 1974.

HUTSCHNECKER, ARNOLD. *The Will to Live*. New York: Cornerstone, 1951.

JAMES, WILLIAM. *Psychology*. New York: World Publishing, 1948.

JAMPOLSKY, GERALD. *Teach Only Love: The Seven Principles of Attitudinal Healing.* New York: Bantam Books, 1983.

JOHNSON, ROBERT. *He: Understanding Masculine Psychology.* New York: Harper & Row, 1977.

———. *She: Understanding Feminine Psychology.* New York: Harper & Row, 1977.

JUNG, CARL. *Modern Man in Search of a Soul.* New York: Harcourt, Brace & Co., 1955.

KRAMER, JOEL. *The Passionate Mind.* Milbrae, Calif.: Celestial Arts, 1973.

KÜBLER-ROSS, ELISABETH. *To Live Until We Say Good-Bye.* Englewood Cliffs, N.J.: Prentice-Hall, 1978.

LAPPÉ, FRANCES. *Diet for a Small Planet.* New York: Random House, 1975.

LESHAN, LAWRENCE. *You Can Fight to Save Your Life: Emotional Factors in the Causation of Cancer.* New York: Evans, 1977.

LEVI, L. *Society, Stress and Disease.* New York: Oxford University Press, 1971.

LEWIS, HOWARD. *Psychosomatics: How Your Emotions Can Damage Your Health.* New York: The Viking Press, 1972.

LINGERMAN, HAL. *The Healing Energies of Music.* Wheaton, Ill.: Theosophical Publishers, 1983.

LOCKE, STEVEN. *Mind and Immunity.* New York: Institute for the Advancement of Health, 1983.

LOWEN, ALEXANDER. *Love and Orgasm.* New York: Macmillan, 1965.

MENNINGER, KARL. *The Vital Balance: The Life Process in Mental Health and Illness.* New York: The Viking Press, 1963.

NEWELL, K. W., ed. *Health by the People.* Geneva: World Health Organization, 1975.

NOUWEN, HENRI. *The Wounded Healer: Ministry in Contemporary Society.* New York: Doubleday, 1979.

NUERNBERGER, P. *Freedom from Stress.* New York: Himalayan International Institute, 1981.

PENFIELD, W. *The Mystery of the Mind.* Princeton, N.J.: Princeton University Press, 1975.

PERCY, WALKER. *Lost in the Cosmos: The Last Self-Help Book.* New York: Farrar, Straus & Giroux, 1984.

PROGOFF, IRA. *The Well and the Cathedral.* New York: Dialog House, 1981.

ROHRLICH, JAY. *Work and Love: The Crucial Balance.* New York: Harmony Books, 1980.

RUSH, ANNE. *Getting Clear.* New York: Random House, 1973.

SATIR, VIRGINIA. *Peoplemaking.* Palo Alto, Calif.: Science and Behavior Books, 1972.

SCHUTZ, WILL. *Profound Simplicity.* New York: Bantam Books, 1979.

SCHWEITZER, ALBERT. *Out of My Life and Thought.* New York: Holt, 1949.

SELBY, JOHN. *Finding Each Other.* Dorset, Eng.: Element Books, 1987 (American distribution by The Great Tradition, San Rafael, Calif.).

————. *The Visual Handbook.* Dorset, Eng.: Element Books, 1988 (American distribution by The Great Tradition, San Rafael, Calif.).

SELYE, HANS. *The Stress of Life.* New York: McGraw-Hill, 1978.

SILVERMAN, S. *Psychological Cues in Forecasting Physical Illness.* New York: Appleton Century, 1970.

INDEX

personal power and, 115, 116
Heartbreak, *see* Grief
Heart disease, 169–71
  Direct Focusing and, 26–27, 29
  inhibited anger and, 32
  love and recovery from, 151, 153
Helplessness, 43
  AIDS and, 174–75
  dependency and, 148
  in hospital, 140, 141
  personal power undermined by, 115
  self-image and, 102
Herb tea, 71
Holistic system of energy centers, 52
Homeostasis, 1–2, 4
  emotional, 33
Honesty, emotional, 67
Hope, xi
Hopelessness, 34, 42–43, 45, 47, 97
  grief and, 42
Hormones:
  growth-stimulating, 4
  personal power and, 114
Hospital:
  guided fantasy while in, 142–49
  eating in, 71–72
  surviving stay in, 138–42
  television in, 77
Human immunodeficiency virus (HIV), 172
Hunger, *see* Passion

Hyperacidity:
  in mouth, 159
  in stomach, 156
Hypnotic suggestion, 61
Hypoglycemia, 161–63
Hypothalamus, xi

Imagination, *see* Fantasies
Impotence, self-image and, 148
Indians, *see* American Indians
Infections:
  cellular behavior in dealing with, 97–98
  chronic, 160–61
  tooth, 159–60, 166, 168
Inhibition of emotions, 32, 34, 45, 55, 64, 66
  diabetes and, 165
Inner child, violation of needs of, 170
Interpersonal needs, 140
Intuitive activation, 127–29

Japan, spiritual tradition of, 127
Jaw muscles, 55
  emotions and, 37
  relaxation of, 18–19, 60, 119
  tension in, 159
Jesus, 151
Joint pains, 29
Joy, xi
  See also Bliss
Juices, 73, 156
Junk food, 74

Kidney infections, 160
Ki energy center, 53